A Life of Control

A Life of Control

Stories of Living with Diabetes

Alan L. Graber, MD

Anne W. Brown, RN, MSN

Kathleen Wolff, RN, MSN

Foreword by Steven G. Gabbe, MD

Vanderbilt University Press

NASHVILLE

© 2010 by Alan L. Graber,
Anne W. Brown, and Kathleen Wolff
Nashville, Tennessee 37235

First printing 2010

This book is printed on acid-free paper
made from 30% post-consumer recycled content.
Manufactured in the United States of America

Library of Congress Cataloging-in-Publication Data

Graber, Alan L. (Alan Lee), 1935–
A life of control : stories of living with diabetes /
Alan L. Graber, Anne W. Brown, Kathleen Wolff ;
foreword by Steven G. Gabbe
p. cm.
Includes bibliographical references and index.
ISBN 978-0-8265-1732-6 (cloth : alk. paper)
ISBN 978-0-8265-1733-3 (pbk. : alk. paper)
1. Diabetes—Popular works.   2. Diabetics—
Family relationships. 3. Self-care, Health.
I. Brown, Anne W., 1952– . II. Wolff, Kathleen, 1953– .
III. Title.
RC660.4.G73 2010
616.4′62—dc22
2009049239

Contents

Foreword

I diagnosed myself to have diabetes mellitus more than four decades ago when I was a medical student. Since then, I have lived every day with diabetes. There haven't been any holidays, three-day weekends, or vacations without diabetes. It hasn't been easy. Yet, with very few exceptions, it has not limited my life in any significant way.

As with any long journey, there have been periods when I thought I was walking up the steepest hill imaginable, periods of smooth sailing, and several detours. A map lets us know where we started, where we are going, and how we can get there. Here are some of the important lessons that have helped me chart my course on my long journey with diabetes mellitus.

First, diabetes is an important part of my life, but it is not me, and it is not my life. I haven't let control of my blood glucose control me. To put it simply, I am more than a blood sugar! As a medical student, I was given the appropriate advice that a career in pathology or radiology might be more compatible with the regular lifestyle that would be best for someone with diabetes. Instead, I chose to go into the subspecialty of high-risk obstetrics or maternal-fetal medicine. I could not have chosen a more demanding field, given its long and irregular hours. Yet, it was the field I was most passionate about, and its patients the ones I most wanted to help, and so I followed my heart.

I have never regretted that decision. I decided to pursue a career in academic medicine that would enable me not only to care for patients but to teach others and conduct research. It has been highly rewarding. I am now privileged to serve as the Senior Vice President for Health Sciences and Chief Executive Officer of the Ohio State University Medical Center, and I still have the opportunity to help others understand what I have learned about diabetes mellitus. Along the way, I have run two marathons and many half-marathons, and with my wife, Dr. Patricia Temple Gabbe, raised four children.

Second, living with diabetes mellitus requires a team effort. It begins with your family, and I could not have done this without the support of my wife and children. Living with diabetes day-to-day also depends on a team of skilled professionals, including physicians, nutritionists, nurse educators, social workers, and pharmacists.

Along the way, I have benefited so much from the care and guidance I have received from my doctors. Dr. Priscilla White of the Joslin Clinic not only taught me how to live with diabetes, but she inspired me to follow in her footsteps, providing care for pregnant women with diabetes and conducting basic and clinical research in this field. At the University of Southern California, Dr. Jorge Mestman told me, "Steve, don't think of diabetes as a disease. Think of it as a condition that you live with. I bet that if you follow your diet, get regular medical care, exercise, and don't smoke, you will be far healthier than most of your friends." That simple message—diabetes as a condition and not a disease—has stayed with me for more than thirty years, and Dr. Mestman was right! At the University of Washington, Dr. Irl Hirsch convinced me that I should try an insulin pump. While I was hesitant at first, I am so appreciative that he recommended this therapy, as it has given me greater flexibility in living with diabetes. At Ohio State, Dr. Sam Cataland has helped me deal with the challenges of exercising and avoiding hypoglycemia.

During the past five years, my colleagues and I have conducted research studies to examine burnout in academic leaders. Risk for burnout can be related to three important factors: demand, control, and support. Living each day with diabetes is certainly demanding, and there are times when, as a patient, you feel that no matter what you do, you have lost control. It is for this reason that support is so important—support from your family, from your friends, and from your health care team.

Third, I have learned so much from my patients over the years. Pregnant women with diabetes are incredibly motivated to do whatever they can to have healthy babies. I have been inspired by their commitment, and it has helped me on my journey with diabetes.

Finally, I have always been an optimist. I recently spoke to our medical students about my life with diabetes, and I called my talk "A Half Full Glass of Lemonade." Because I work at one of the leading academic medical centers in the country, and because each day I hear about the advances in research and patient care that are being made, I am more optimistic now than I have ever been. When I began my long journey with diabetes, there were few insulins available, and we used glass syringes and needles that had to be sharpened. So much has changed! We have a variety of new insulin analogues that help us live more flexible lives, new oral medications for individuals with type 2 diabetes mellitus, portable blood glucose meters that keep getting smaller and faster, glycosylated hemoglobin measurements to give us overviews of our control in previous months, and insulin pumps that can help us adjust to even the most hectic and erratic work schedules and lifestyles. Continuous glucose sensors have recently become available; in the coming years, I am confident we will see sensors talking to pumps, effectively creating an artificial pancreas. And then there also remains the hope that continued research in stem cell biology and immunology will lead to interventions that can prevent and cure diabetes.

It is my hope that wherever you are on your journey with diabetes, my comments and the stories in this important book will make your trip just a bit easier.

Steven G. Gabbe, MD

Preface

There are many perspectives to the story of diabetes: those of doctors, nurses, pharmaceutical investigators, molecular biologists, behavioral scientists, and epidemiologists studying a worldwide epidemic. But the most significant perspectives are those of the individuals whose lives are involved with this illness. The history of an illness is inseparable from the life being lived around it—the person's family, his work, his world. Diabetes happens in a life that already has a story. The purpose of these personal narratives is to situate the diabetes experience within patients' lives and the meaning of those lives.

Both the patient and the health care provider have stories about their relationship. Their stories are intertwined but not always harmonious. The encounters between the two are a significant part of a patient's life, but not necessarily the most important part. These narratives offer both patients and providers opportunities to reflect upon the richness and tension of such interactions.

While we have provided some information about diabetes—at least enough to allow the reader to understand the significance of each story—we have not intended to make this a textbook on diabetes or a self-care manual for patients. There are many excellent resources for self-care both in print and on the Internet, some of which are listed at the end of this book.

Unless otherwise noted, I (Dr. Graber) am the narrator of this book. It is based not only on my forty years of practice as an endocrinologist, but also on that of the two nurse practitioners whose compassion and skill have aided me and my patients. Anne Brown and Kathleen Wolff were classmates in the nurse practitioner program at Vanderbilt University School of Nursing. After joining me, they became certified as diabetes educators and as advanced diabetes management nurse practitioners. While I focused on diagnosis and scientific treatment, they brought to my practice the perspective of a different discipline, one more concerned with helping and caring. I learned from them that it took more than the knowledge of a medical specialist to control diabetes. For the past twenty-five years, the three of us have worked together on a daily basis, first in private practice and later at the Vanderbilt Eskind Diabetes Center.

To encompass the scope of diabetes, this book is divided into sections that are defined by the main elements of diabetes control. The first section consists of stories in which patient self-determination was the critical factor. Some responses led to successful efforts to control diabetes, while others were ineffective or even destructive. The second section describes the role of the family from the viewpoints of patients, parents, and spouses. The third section demonstrates instances where the social situation was the most influential factor. In the fourth section, the complex interaction between the patient and clinician is illustrated. The Conclusion focuses on the prevention of diabetes. The lives of patients with diabetes defy precise categorization, and therefore many stories in this book contain themes that overlap across multiple sections.

Conversations with our patients with diabetes usually revolve around the problems of control. "I try to keep my diabetes under control" and "I've never been in control" are statements we hear every week. Many of our patients have been told by another physician, "I'm referring you to a specialist, because your diabetes is out of control."

An individual's acquaintance with diabetes largely depends upon the type of diabetes present. Type 1 and type 2 share the name "diabetes" and the potential health risks that result from prolonged elevation of the blood sugar (such as eventual damage to the eyes, kidneys, and heart) but little other common ground. Type 1 diabetes refers to the destruction of insulin-producing cells in the pancreas. Formerly called "juvenile diabetes" because it most often begins during childhood or adolescence, type 1 diabetes can begin at any age. If the condition is not recognized and treated adequately with insulin injections, it can lead to coma and death. Michael Bliss's book *The Discovery of Insulin* describes the critical importance of insulin treatment in saving the lives of patients with type 1 diabetes: "The discovery of insulin at the University of Toronto in 1921–1922 was one of the most dramatic events in the history of disease. Those who watched the first starved, sometimes comatose, diabetics receive insulin and return to life saw one of the genuine miracles of modern medicine."[1]

Type 1 diabetes affects about one million people in the United

States, but it constitutes less than 5 percent of the total population of patients with diabetes. In contrast, type 2 diabetes, now epidemic in scope because of the increasing prevalence of obesity, is the fastest growing health problem both nationally and globally. An estimated one of every three Americans will have this disease by the year 2050. Today, about one of every three children and adolescents is overweight. As a result, the incidence of type 2 diabetes is increasing rapidly among adolescents, an age group in which it was virtually unknown a few decades earlier.[2]

In type 2 diabetes, the body produces reduced amounts of insulin, but resistance to the effect of insulin is an important feature and begins many years before high blood sugar appears. Type 2 diabetes is more likely to affect people who are older, and most individuals who develop type 2 diabetes are overweight. Sometimes patients with type 2 diabetes have few or no symptoms, and they may experience one of its consequences (such as a heart attack) before it is discovered. If there are no symptoms, usually the physician first suggests lifestyle changes, with instructions pertaining to diet and exercise. Since lifestyle practices have become fixed by the time these patients develop diabetes, changing their eating and exercise habits poses great challenges. If lifestyle changes do not result in normalization of blood sugar levels, pills to lower blood sugar are added next. Most patients ultimately require treatment with insulin, since pills become insufficient as insulin production declines.

The daily and consuming diligence required of patients and families with type 1 diabetes is seldom practiced by those with type 2 diabetes. Some people with type 2 diabetes do not even consider diabetes a serious disease. For example, among those over age sixty, where as many as 20 percent may have diabetes, they hardly consider themselves different. Control of mild type 2 diabetes with no symptoms has few immediate rewards. Controlling diabetes at that point can be compared to fastening one's seat belt. There is no positive feedback—just the hypothetical avoidance of frightening results in the future.

For the diabetes health professional, control means maintaining the level of glucose in the blood as close to normal as possible. To complicate matters, blood glucose levels fluctuate constantly, increasing after eating or with stress, decreasing during exercise. Almost every event of daily living—every meal, every activity, every illness, every injury or surgery, and even every emotional change—affects blood glucose levels. In a person without diabetes, one whose pancreas functions normally, adjustments in insulin levels are accomplished automatically. But in a person with diabetes, these adjustments do not occur automatically. They must be initiated by the patient.

The ability of a person to monitor the level of his blood sugar has been one of the most important advances in diabetes care. He pricks his finger with a spring-loaded lancet to obtain a drop of blood that is placed on a chemically sensitive strip and inserted into a portable battery-operated glucose monitor about the size of a small cellular telephone. Within seconds, the blood glucose level is displayed on a screen. Most patients with type 1 diabetes and many with type 2 diabetes who use insulin are instructed to test themselves four times daily—before meals and at bedtime—and to use the results to determine their doses of insulin.

But control of diabetes is much more than monitoring the blood glucose. Since the major complications of diabetes are also affected by blood pressure and the level of cholesterol in the blood, adequate control of diabetes includes control of these problems as well. As a starter, persons with diabetes must pursue the ABCs of diabetes control: "A" refers to the A1c test, "B" refers to blood pressure, and "C" refers to blood cholesterol level.

The A1c laboratory test indicates the average blood glucose for the preceding two or three months. A1c levels are related to the risk for long-term diabetes complications. The recommended target for persons with diabetes is less than 7 percent. Fewer than a third of patients with diabetes have achieved this goal.[3] The measured A1c result is increasingly being reported as the estimated average glucose value (eAG), which simplifies its interpretation both for health care providers and for patients.[4]

Some of the long-term complications of diabetes are more closely related to blood pressure than to blood sugar. The target level of blood pressure for patients with diabetes is below 130/80 if it can be safely achieved. Such levels can be accomplished with a single antihypertensive drug in some, but many patients require three or more different types of antihypertensive drugs to achieve this goal.[5]

Prevention of heart attacks, the main cause of death in persons with diabetes, is more closely related to the level of LDL cholesterol (the "bad" cholesterol) in the blood than to blood sugar. The recommended target for LDL cholesterol in the general adult population is below 130 mg/dl, but in most patients with diabetes, because of the increased risk of heart attack, the recommended target level is below

100 mg/dl, and even lower if possible.[6] If a diet low in saturated fats doesn't achieve the desired level of LDL cholesterol, a patient may then be prescribed a lipid-lowering drug (usually a statin). All persons with diabetes are also advised to take a low dose of aspirin daily to prevent the formation of blood clots.

The damage inflicted by cigarette smoking can undermine all the benefits of good blood sugar, cholesterol, and blood pressure control. Cigarette smoking can never be a part of adequate diabetes control. Control of diabetes also includes monitoring for early signs of complications and treating them to limit progression; pre-pregnancy planning for women with childbearing potential; and addressing depression and other mental health disorders.

The health professional's view of diabetes control includes all the above-mentioned laboratory tests, exams, medications, and counseling. For the patient, this view of control may appear complex, time-consuming, and expensive. Clinicians' warnings about the complications of diabetes may seem overly grim to patients unwilling to face the possibilities of kidney disease, blindness, or amputation, particularly when such complications are unlikely to occur until many years into the future. Many people with diabetes look and feel healthy most of the time, but in diabetes, the background and foreground of health and sickness constantly shade into each other. The patient views himself as a person whose life is complicated by diabetes, not as a professional patient. The health professional's view of diabetes control is only a window into the many dimensions of a life with diabetes, which will be illustrated in the following collection of patient narratives.

The stories in this book are actual accounts from the lives of patients we have known. Most are based on taped interviews. Quotes indicate a patient's actual words. Almost all patients described herein have been given pseudonyms. In some cases, we have changed additional details to assure anonymity and confidentiality. A few have asked that their real names be used. Medical terms are defined in the Glossary.

A Life of Control

PART I

The Patient in Control

At first glance, control of diabetes would appear to be directed by the clinician and implemented by the patient. In no other disease does the patient assume so much of the responsibility for its daily treatment. But only a portion of a patient's life concerns are related to the clinical problem of diabetes, and the clinician oversees only that portion. One of the limitations of the clinician–patient relationship is the patient's desire for autonomy. For some patients, the constraints imposed by diabetes, translated to them via the clinician, are viewed at least subconsciously as attempts to take over control of their lives.

While interviewing patients for this book, we heard both the stories of diabetes and the stories of the people living with it. We identified suffering, tension, conflict, and defiance in the lives of our patients. We witnessed heroism in some, despair in others.

Strong feelings were expressed in such statements as "I can't hand over control of my life to my doctor" and "my doctor may know diabetes, but he doesn't understand me." Independence in the control of diabetes was exemplified by the notion, "I'll control diabetes so it won't control me." The continuum of the patient's struggle for autonomy extended from frank rebellion against the physician's advice and rejection of any authority to instances of remarkable self-motivation.

The narratives in this section emphasize the role of patient self-determination as the prime element of control. Many patients pursued their own ideas of diabetes control. In some cases, the clinician–patient relationship had only limited influence on diabetes control. The voice of the clinician was acknowledged, but the voice of the patient predominated.

CHAPTER 1

To Hell with Diabetes

Nikki developed diabetes at age fifteen. She related, "It was OK at first, but as I got older and started going out, I didn't want to test my blood sugar or take insulin—it was inconvenient. I was the only teenager I knew who had diabetes. I felt fine physically, but I cried a lot. Why did it happen to me? I wasn't depressed, I was angry. If I could have given it to someone, I would have."

In her high school courses, she made all As and Bs. Her parents were both professionals in the field of education, and she stated, "They didn't want to see a C. I did my homework. I was a cheerleader for two years. I had the lead female part in the senior play. Teenagers rebel about everything, but I wasn't rebellious. Sometimes I just wanted to give up, forget about school, forget about going out, forget about diabetes." And that's exactly what she did.

Between the ages of sixteen and twenty-one, throughout high school and the first two years of college, she was hospitalized at least once a year for diabetic ketoacidosis (DKA). The major acute complication of type 1 diabetes, DKA is characterized by vomiting, dehydration, and eventually coma and death. Sometimes it is the initial manifestation of type 1 diabetes, occurring before the patient or family realizes that diabetes is present. In individuals with established diabetes, an infection or other acute illness can precipitate DKA, but when it occurs repeatedly, omission of insulin is usually the cause.

Why would an intelligent young woman repeatedly quit taking her insulin injections, knowing that she would end up in the hospital and might even die? We held a medical conference to discuss our difficulties in caring for patients like Nikki, most of whom were young women. The doctors and nurses who attended the conference concluded that in most cases, the patients must have intentionally omitted their insulin injections, although few admitted it. One attendee quoted a patient who had acknowledged, "I didn't take my insulin shots after arguments with my mother, my boyfriend, and a girl at work. I knew I would get sick and start vomiting in a few hours, and even if I lost consciousness, someone would take me to the emergency room, and they'd put me in the hospital." The patient understood her disease perfectly and knew that only she had control over her insulin injections. She knew that she could allow the development of DKA whenever she chose to, and that no hospital could refuse to treat a readily curable acute medical emergency.

When her mother had suggested that she see a psychologist, Nikki had replied, "If you make me go, I'll just sit there and not say anything." Then, at age twenty-one, she didn't take her insulin for a month. She told me that she had said to herself, *To hell with diabetes. I was free of insulin, free of sticking my finger, free of anything negative from diabetes. I was determined that nothing would happen to me.*" She stated that she had had the usual symptoms of diabetes—thirst, drinking lots of water, tiredness, and the loss of thirty-five pounds—but she had continued to function and thought her body had adjusted to high blood sugar.

Finally, one day she got sick at her boyfriend's house; she couldn't get her breath and felt she was going to pass out. "I told him to call my dad, not my mom. Momma would give it to me straight, and I didn't want to hear anything straight. I wanted it sugarcoated." By the time she was admitted to the hospital with severe DKA, she was in a coma.

Every medical student knows that if DKA is not treated, death can occur. Since the condition results from insulin deficiency, the basis of treatment is relatively straightforward: provide insulin and restore the several liters of fluid that have been lost. During the previous generation of medical students, a popular professor at Vanderbilt had a dramatic way of teaching his first-year physiology students about DKA. He would divide the class into teams of four students and issue each team a laboratory rat. Then he would instruct the students to surgically remove the pancreas from their rat. Without a pancreas, the rat would lack insulin, developing DKA and dying within a day or so unless it received treatment. He taught the students to monitor the level of sugar and other chemicals in blood drawn from the rat's tail. The students would deliver insulin and fluids to the rat, trying to cure the DKA and keep the rat alive. This was the students' first opportunity to stay up all night at the bedside and try to save a life. Despite their best efforts, some of the rats died, but those teams of students who understood the abnormal physiology and its treatment succeeded in keeping their rat alive for several days, finally ending the process because they were exhausted. They could boast to their classmates that they were destined to be great rat doctors.

Nikki received excellent medical treatment in the hospital, and the DKA resolved, though she remained in a coma for twenty hours. When she finally regained consciousness, she was frightened. "The coma was something the doctors had warned me about. If I went into a coma again, it might not be for twenty hours, it might be for twenty days. I thought it was time for me to straighten up."

Nikki was referred to a clinical psychologist. This time she said, "OK, I'll go, but if I don't get anything out of it, I'm not going back."

But the psychologist was extremely helpful. "When they brought the psychologist in, I got vibes from her that she understood—that she was compassionate and willing to help. I could sense she knew what she was doing and she would do anything in her power to get me to understand that diabetes was part of me and wasn't going away. I could feel a lot of things being lifted from me. It was easier talking to someone who didn't know me; it was easier for me to get everything off my shoulders without worrying about her feelings being hurt or my feelings being hurt from what she would say back to me. She was a confidence builder."

Nikki appreciated the fact that the psychologist understood diabetes but never told her what she had to do. She related, "The psychologist asked how I thought my parents would cope with losing me. From then on, I took every insulin shot. I did better than I ever had. I thought about how my loss would affect other people. I knew my mom would go ballistic. I didn't want to cause my mom more pain than she had already felt. When the psychologist gave me the chance to step out of my shoes and into someone else's, that was my first rude awakening."

When I interviewed Nikki for this book, she was a twenty-six-year-old grad student and five years past her last hospitalization. I asked her pointedly, "When you omitted insulin, what was the underlying reason? Were you trying to harm yourself? Were you trying to get attention?"

She replied, "I wasn't trying to kill myself, and I wasn't trying to get anybody's attention. I knew the consequences. I was just burnt out from having diabetes. I didn't care. I hated testing my blood sugar, and I still do. It only takes five seconds, and it doesn't actually hurt. I honestly don't know what it is about that sticking the finger thing, but I just hate it with a passion."

I pressed further: "Didn't it bother you going into the hospital every year?" I was appalled by her answer: "It only bothered me because I missed my extracurricular activities while I was in the hospital. My friends were doing things that I didn't want to miss, like going to football games or pep rallies. The doctors told me that it could be worse the next time, but I thought they were just using a scare tactic. Every time it was the same: they would give me IVs and insulin, I'd go home in a few days, and I would start taking my insulin again. Making up all that work from school didn't bother me."

Approximately 100,000 hospitalizations for DKA occur in this country annually. Though DKA can usually be treated effectively in a modern hospital, the mortality rate is still considerable. Nikki was risking her life every time it occurred.

CHAPTER 2

I Threw Away the Sugar Bowl

Four days after she was diagnosed with type 2 diabetes, Peggy was referred by her primary care physician to a diabetes nurse practitioner. "Kathleen calmed me down that first day," Peggy recounted. "She gave me hope, she gave me knowledge, she knew what she was doing. She reached over and touched me and said, 'You can control this, and if you do, there's a good chance you won't have to go on insulin.' The thing that scared me was going on insulin. It wasn't the fear of shots. I didn't want to become dependent on anything again. I had had acute respiratory distress syndrome [ARDS] eleven years ago and had been dependent on oxygen for two years. I made up my mind that day to control the blood sugar, whatever it took."

Kathleen remembers that "Peggy's blood sugar had been extremely high. In a different setting, with a different clinician, insulin would have been prescribed, but she had already begun to change her eating habits, she had faithfully taken the medication prescribed by her primary care doctor, and her blood sugar had already decreased. I made the decision to give her the chance to control her blood sugar without insulin injections, although I was not convinced that she could succeed. I insisted that she contact me daily to report her blood sugar and general progress."

Peggy said:

I went home, threw away the sugar bowl, and replaced it with Splenda. Then I cleaned out the refrigerator and the cabinets and never looked back. I had no control when I had ARDS, but I could breathe now. I felt I could have some control over what I did with diabetes. It would take a major life change to do it, and this was it.

I didn't know what I could eat that night; I had to get a plan. I got on the Internet and looked up diets for diabetes. Then I drove to the bookstore and got books about diets for diabetes. I called a friend with diabetes. I got through the first few days by just going from one meal to another. At 289 pounds, I knew that I had caused diabetes by being overweight. My sleep apnea, arthritis, and other health problems could be improved with weight loss. Once, in grad school, I had lost ninety pounds and kept it off about five years. I woke up one day and had gained it all back. Now, losing weight wasn't my number one goal, it was controlling my blood sugar.

She learned quickly. She limited her carbohydrate intake to forty-five grams per meal. Peggy supplied the details:

For the first few months, it took me hours to grocery shop. Nothing went into my grocery cart or my mouth that wasn't in that little book of carbohydrates. I bought scales and measuring cups. I bought smaller plates and bowls. Before diabetes, I would start answering phone calls as part of my job as soon as I got up; then I would be starving and eat a big lunch. Now I plan my meals. I eat three meals a day including a good breakfast; turkey bacon is my favorite. I didn't dare go to a restaurant for three months. I didn't trust myself. I didn't eat any pasta whatsoever; now pasta is sometimes a side dish, never a main meal. I eat lots of salads. I bought a new car with a cooler between the seats, and when I travel on business, I put snacks and lunch in the cooler. I don't look at it as a diet; it is what I have to do to control my blood sugar. It was very hard in the beginning, but now it's second nature.

During the first month after the diagnosis of diabetes, Peggy lost six pounds, and another six pounds the second month. She noted that the improvement in her blood sugar levels occurred as soon as she modified her diet—much more quickly than the loss of weight. By four months, she had lost twenty-five pounds. Her A1c had fallen to 5.1 percent, within the normal range. The liver enzymes indicating excess fat in her liver normalized. After a year, she had lost seventy pounds and had been able to stop her diabetes pills. "Coming off oral medicines meant a lot to me; it meant I didn't need anything external to control diabetes. I know if I don't watch my diet, those blood sugars will go back up, so I don't have a choice."

Peggy described how she dealt with some of her trials. "Thanksgiving came six months after my diagnosis of diabetes. I panicked. What was I going to do when the family got together? My family has great recipes. We sit down and talk to one another with food. I decided to eat one tablespoonful of everything. For most things, that was all I really wanted, but when the pies came out, it was hard. I got the thinnest sliver of both my mom's pecan pie and my grandmother's pumpkin pie. The next day I went back to my regular eating, and everything was OK. Next I worried about Christmas, but I used the same tactics. This Easter we didn't have the traditional meal that we have always had. We changed it. It was almost like betraying my grandmother. We had a spiral-baked ham, cut thinner than the hams we used to bake, and we had fresh green beans instead of baked beans. We did have a bowl of potato salad, but I took only one tablespoon."

I inquired of Peggy what accounted for her success. She said, "I was raised with the attitude that you do whatever you have to do. My mother was a single mom who raised three girls. She always worked two or three jobs. I watched her do the impossible. Nothing ever came easily for her or for me, and I had to work for everything. When I looked at diabetes, I felt I had two choices. I could be a diabetic on insulin, or I could be a diabetic who controlled it."

I asked Peggy if she sets goals for herself. "I do," she replied, "but I don't want to box myself in. I would like to lose another thirty-five pounds, but I won't commit to any specific weight goals. It would have been too overwhelming to aim to lose seventy pounds. I set small goals. If I eat the way I should to control my blood sugar, I'll probably continue to lose some weight."

As we completed the interview, Peggy added with a smile, "One of my goals is to control diabetes so I won't end up in your office. Nothing personal."

Eighty percent of people with type 2 diabetes are overweight. When type 2 diabetes is diagnosed in an overweight person, medical professionals always recommend weight loss. Weight loss decreases resistance to insulin and almost always improves the patient's blood sugar levels.

Sometimes weight loss improves diabetes control so much that no medications are needed, and blood sugar can be controlled just by attention to food intake and weight.

Control of type 2 diabetes requires the same dedication, planning, and attention to detail as type 1 diabetes. Whereas in type 1 diabetes the focus is on the proper dose of insulin, in type 2 diabetes the same vigorous attention must be focused on controlling food intake. In each situation, the medical professional plays a supporting role, as Kathleen did with Peggy, but the decisive factors are the individual's motivation and follow-through.

CHAPTER 3

Running for My Life

Kathleen has known Dottie as a friend for twenty-five years and even played the harp at her wedding. She recalls her shock when she walked into the treatment room in her role as a nurse practitioner and saw Dottie receiving intravenous fluids. "People were hovering over her," Kathleen relates. "When I looked at her, she was withered and thin, thin, thin. She looked worn and exhausted. It was hard to reconcile, because I had not seen the progression from powerfully fit to gaunt. I had to adjust in a split second, for I didn't want her to see me gasp, but that's what I did inside. I wasn't worried about her safety at that moment. I knew that as soon as she got IV fluids and insulin in her body, she'd be on her way back to 100 percent. She had so much experience taking on challenges, things that would intimidate other people. She had worked as a nurse in the emergency room, in the intensive care unit, and as a life flight nurse in a helicopter. I had to process the fact that my friend Dottie—this vibrant, strong, athletic, adventuresome woman—now suddenly had type 1 diabetes."

Dottie recalls, "I was training for my first marathon, and it just wasn't happening for me. I had felt tired for six months, lethargic all the time, even worse when exercising. During a sixteen-mile training run, I'd have to stop and walk after three or four miles. I had always done well on the hills, but my running buddies were having to slow down for me. It just didn't add up. I attributed it to stress. Within the past six months, there had been a deluge of stress. First my mother-in-law had died, then two weeks later my mother died. A week after that, my sister was found to have untreatable cancer. I was working fifty to sixty hours a week in the operating room training to be a nurse anesthetist. I didn't have time to figure it out. I just kept running. Running was supposed to make it better, but it didn't."

Running in the August heat in Nashville, Dottie began to pass copious amounts of urine and to experience intense thirst. "I lost eighteen pounds," Dottie recounts. "The lady who gave me massages said I was very bony. I couldn't get enough to eat. I had a vaginal yeast infection for six months, intractable to all treatment. My vision changed, and that was the worst. As a nurse, I didn't diagnose myself with diabetes, but neither did my gynecologist nor my eye doctor."

After two weeks of the excessive urination and thirst, she saw her primary care provider, who performed extensive tests. After the examination, she was so hungry that she ate a chocolate chip cookie. Then she drove to Belle Meade Boulevard for a run. "I had to stop twice during the six-mile run. I thought I might faint. Then each time I felt better while walking. It was a terrible run, but I finished it. The next day my primary care provider called me and said my blood sugar was 600 mg/dl, that I should go to the diabetes clinic and start insulin immediately."

Upon arrival in the diabetes clinic, Dottie was profoundly dehydrated. She was given intravenous fluids and started on insulin treatment. I was the physician in the clinic and met Dottie that day. She told me that she had run about twenty half-marathons, and that in four weeks she was scheduled to run a full 26.2 mile marathon in California with her best friend from Montana. The reservations were made and paid for. I was familiar with the obsession—I'm a runner myself—but I didn't think marathon training was medically safe for Dottie until her diabetes was under control and she had regained her weight. I recommended she not run for at least two weeks, though walking and easy swimming would be fine. I feared that she would not follow my advice.

"I didn't run for two weeks after the diagnosis of diabetes, as Dr. Graber instructed," Dottie says. "When I started running again, my blood sugars were still in the mid-200 range, but I felt fine. I realized that there was no way I could run a full marathon. I decided to settle for the half-marathon, and I did fine in the race in California. I ran nine-minute miles, feeling great. A few weeks later, I transitioned to an insulin pump."

Two years after the onset of diabetes, Dottie says, "I've always been a strong swimmer. We have a pool at home, and I swim almost every day. I usually run three to five days a week, depending on my work schedule. The shortest run is about thirty minutes, the longer ones up to 1½ hours. I do more if I'm training for a half-marathon."

Dottie states that she always eats food containing carbohydrates about an hour before any type of training or competition, knowing that her blood sugar will be a little high when she starts, and expecting it to drop as she exercises:

> Swimming in a pool is fine. If I feel that my blood sugar is getting low, I take some Gatorade, which is always at the side of the pool. For me, the first symptoms of low blood sugar are lethargy and a feeling of floating. It's hard to pick up these symptoms while swimming, so I have to take precautions if I plan to swim a mile in a lake. I keep a packet of GlucoBurst glucose gel with me. It contains fifteen grams of glucose in a flexible foil package that can fit in the palm of my hand. The package is easy to store in a pocket and easy to use. I just tear it at the notch and squeeze the contents into my mouth and swallow. I can stop and take the glucose while treading water. After any workout, I always check my blood sugar, and it's usually between 90 and 120 mg/dl [normal].
>
> Before a long run, I take off my insulin pump, to avoid low blood sugar. I keep my glucagon injection and my insulin pump in a cooler in the car. I store Gatorade in the trunk. When I run, I always carry Gatorade and glucose tablets or GlucoBurst, so I have two forms of sugar on me at all times. These are the little important things that you learn.
>
> I did a triathlon a few weeks ago. In a triathlon you can spend a lot of time in the transitions [between swimming and cycling, and between cycling and running]. I debated whether to check my blood sugar during the transitions, but I felt so well I decided not to bother checking it. I just took another packet of GlucoBurst. During the run, I could feel my blood sugar dropping a little, but I had some Gatorade, and it was no problem.

When asked how her current training routine differs from that before the onset of diabetes, Dottie says, "I do as much now as I did before, but it just doesn't feel as good—it's not as much fun. Biking and swimming seem easier than running. Comparing it to five years ago, before I started anesthesia school, I have to start more slowly, and my times are a little slower. I don't know if it's my age [forty-six] or the fact that I'm perimenopausal, but maybe I still don't have the right match between sugar and insulin. I'm still learning. For conditioning purposes, I'm making myself run during the hot part of the day. I ran about an hour today when it was almost ninety degrees. Tomorrow is Sunday, and my husband and I will do a twenty-five-mile bicycle ride."

Dottie describes a six-day backpacking trip with her husband in the Teton Mountains. "We hiked about six hours a day at high altitude, so it was pretty strenuous. While walking, I decreased the insulin rate in my pump by 50 percent and drank lots of Gatorade. The first day I checked my blood sugar frequently. After that, I just checked it four times a day, and everything worked out perfectly. When we got to our campsite for the evening, I increased the insulin rate to normal. I had been warned that the blood sugar could drop to low levels for up to twenty-four hours after strenuous exercise, particularly during the night. I awakened and checked my blood sugar in the tent about two a.m. each night. Of course I brought along extra insulin and supplies for my pump. Sometimes heat weakens the strength of my insulin, but I wrapped the insulin bottles and kept them deep in my backpack. With these precautions, the environment didn't seem to affect it. I did great on the trip and had no problems with diabetes."

Diabetes hasn't prevented Dottie from doing what she loves, but she understands the planning and preparation required to do it safely.

The Diabetes Exercise and Sports Association (www.diabetes-exercise .org) is a valuable resource for any athlete with diabetes interested in sports competition. It has three thousand members, conducts frequent conferences, and publishes a quarterly newsletter. The organization was started in 1985 by Paula Harper, a marathon runner who felt she needed more guidance about managing her insulin during exercise. While running a marathon in Phoenix, Arizona, she wore on her back the words "I run on insulin." She currently is a nurse diabetes educator at the Veterans Administration Hospital in Nashville, Tennessee.

CHAPTER 4

A High Price for Weight Loss

"The only way I can control my weight is to deliberately un-control my diabetes," Rosa confessed. A registered nurse with nineteen years' experience with her own diabetes, she knew what she was talking about. She was using an insulin pump—the most advanced method of taking insulin. She programmed its rate of insulin infusion to control her blood sugar to near-normal levels, but only before meals. She knew that when she ate, she would need an extra burst of insulin to prevent the expected post-meal rise in blood sugar. When she omitted these extra bursts of insulin with her meals, a large portion of the sugar in the digested food would spill over into her urine. In this manner, she could eat as much as she wanted, including sweets, and just allow the extra calories to be excreted.

"I was twenty-three, at a university in Puerto Rico studying nursing, when I was found to have diabetes. My mom has twelve siblings, and seven of the twelve have diabetes. I have three brothers, and two have diabetes. I cannot tell you how many of my fifty first cousins have diabetes," Rosa said. Rosa and her family have type 2 diabetes, which is two to three times more frequent in Puerto Ricans than in non-Hispanic whites.

"I weighed 130 when diabetes appeared, and that's a lot if you are 4'11". In college I gained so much weight. The doctor told me that if I lost the weight, the diabetes would go away, and he put me on a diet. I didn't take it too seriously. I graduated that May and started working the next week on a medical-surgical floor. I was very busy. Getting up early and working, I did lose all the extra weight, and my sugar was OK."

After Rosa moved to Nashville, she got a job as a hospital nurse. Soon after, she regained the weight she had lost, and her blood sugar increased again. She needed insulin for control. "Running late, I would forget my insulin. I got married and became pregnant. You [Dr. Gra-ber] said something about the insulin pump."

Rosa described her struggles with her weight:

> Our food is so starchy. I remember growing up, I would have a plate of rice with mashed potatoes. I didn't have diabetes then; I was always 100 pounds. It was always starch and chicken and dessert. Our vegetables are starchy, too: corn, yucca, malanga. We have a great dish that my ma used to make. It's all this starchy food boiled together with olive oil. It's great, but it's heavy.
>
> I married a Cuban. My husband loves to cook, and he's good at it. When he's worked on a dish and serves it, he wants to be sure you like it. The way you show him you like it is to eat more. If I say, "I don't want any more," he'll say, "Oh, you didn't like it? Why, how come you didn't like it?" And he'll say, "Just have a little bit more. Let me have your plate." It's so good that you eat and eat, even if you're full.
>
> My mother-in-law will call, and my husband says, "Yeah, Mom called. She's cooking tonight, so we're going over." Her cooking is unbelievable. I try to eat just a little bit of rice, a little bit of beans and starchy veggies, but I go back for seconds. It's my fault, but it's hard to say no. We get together with family, with brothers and sisters-in-law, and it's all about food.

Rosa said, "When I was pregnant, I started taking care of myself. You told me, 'Rosa, your blood glucose needs to be between 70 and 120 mg/dl to have a healthy baby.' It was. I did get pre-eclampsia, but my baby was fine the whole time." I said, "Rosa, you should be pregnant more often—you took such good care of yourself then."

During pregnancy, Rosa was compulsive in her diabetes care, but after the pregnancy, her difficulties recurred:

> I'm a nurse and I know how to take care of diabetes. You should see me when I talk to my patients about diabetes. "This is about carbs, and if you do this and you do that, your sugar will be in better control." It sounds hypocritical that I tell them to do that and I don't do it myself. Taking care of it isn't so bad or hard, and I have done it sometimes. I do it right for a few weeks, and

it's fine. I know I can live like that, but something always happens. I fall off the wagon. I know how alcoholics feel.

I love my job. I have worked in the operating room, in the medical intensive care unit, on the bone marrow transplant service, and now in the cardiac catheterization lab. My job is hard. It is case after case, and we go, go, go. Sometimes I grab peanut butter and crackers for lunch. I can't stop and test my blood sugar. We say we need to slow down, but if we do, we will work until 8 or 9 p.m.

Rosa had started the maneuver of omitting insulin and allowing uncontrolled diabetes to control her weight when she had gained several pounds. Using this trick, she had already lost twelve pounds without the necessity of dieting.

Rosa readily acknowledged what she had been doing. "Yes, I have been doing that to lose weight for almost a year. I know that as soon as my blood sugar is high, I will pee and get rid of fluid and lots of sugar. Then I will lose weight. I know it isn't healthy. I'm losing weight and still eating cake and candy, but I'm killing myself and my kidneys and my eyes, causing all the complications that go with diabetes."

"You're losing weight because almost half of the calories you consume in your food are ending up in the urine. Wouldn't it be healthier for you if you just threw half of your food into the toilet?" I asked.

Omitting insulin and using uncontrolled diabetes to lose weight has been called "diabulimia." Some of the young women who have tried it have been hospitalized with life-threatening emergencies.

It is well known that uncontrolled diabetes can lead to weight loss. When we evaluate our patients in the clinic, the presence of recent weight loss is sure to get our attention and almost always indicates the need for more intensive diabetes treatment to lower the blood sugar.

CHAPTER 5

I Refuse to View Myself as Sick

David, a cardiologist, was forty-five years old when he discovered that he had type 1 diabetes. Five years later, when asked about his feelings at the time of diagnosis, he replies, "I felt like I had received a death sentence. I was devastated. I did not believe that this could happen to me. It took a few months to get over the depression that came along with it."

It didn't take long for him to start dealing with it, however. Within two weeks, David was wearing an insulin pump and was trying to keep his blood sugar levels as close to normal as possible. "It was no decision for me," he explains. "I was immediately committed to tight control, which was consistent with all my preexisting concepts of health. I had given up red meat thirty years before. I would never have dreamed of using tobacco or drugs or anything that would impair my health. I realized that my brain would have to substitute for my pancreas."

David learned the details of how to control diabetes from an experienced nurse practitioner at the Vanderbilt Diabetes Center. "I view her as my lifesaver," he says, recounting how she taught him to program his pump, insert the insulin infusion needle under his skin, count carbohydrates, and strategize the timing of insulin, meals, and exercise, not only for standard work days but for weekends and travel.

David relates his perception of diabetes before his own diagnosis: "I considered diabetes a scourge. Because of my own professional experiences with patients with diabetes, I despised the disease. As a cardiologist, I had seen the coronary arteries of people with diabetes. I knew what they looked like inside."

The nurse tried to convince David that degenerative complications—including vascular abnormalities in the heart, kidneys, and eyes—were not inevitable if he could maintain near-normal control of his blood sugar levels. She presented to him the experience of numerous patients with type 1 diabetes who had survived over fifty years without any significant complications.[1] For the first few years, he kept a detailed record of every blood sugar reading, meal, and exercise session. He faxed the record weekly to his nurse practitioner, who analyzed it and made suggestions. He now considers those weekly reports a necessary exercise in learning how to self-manage his diabetes.

David considers the frequency of blood sugar monitoring the key. He checks his fingerstick blood sugar an average of fifteen times each day—virtually every hour while awake—including before and after every meal and exercise session, and at bedtime. Several times a week, he also checks it in the middle of the night. His slogan is that by frequent monitoring—what he calls "constant vigilance"—he will never be "too high or too low for too long." His average blood sugar is essentially the same as that of people without diabetes.

At the onset of his diabetes, David had been counseled that he wouldn't have to change his lifestyle to cope with diabetes, but with his emphasis on preventing high blood sugar, he has found that not to be true for him. "There are so many variables every day. Since I am so committed to tight control, it affects every waking moment. For example, I have to choose times carefully for eating and working out, and I've had to decrease the amount of carbohydrates in my diet, even while using the insulin pump."

He often eats the same thing day after day just because he knows how much insulin to use for it. As a result of his intense efforts to avoid high blood sugar, he has low blood sugar a few hours after breakfast virtually daily, requiring a snack in the middle of the morning. None of the episodes of low blood sugar are severe or require assistance from others, but sometimes he must excuse himself temporarily while examining a patient or during a meeting.

"Diabetes affects almost every aspect of my life," he explains. Initially, he considered changing careers, because the demands of taking calls at night or on weekends created situations difficult to anticipate. "I need safeguards and predictability," he says.

"It was a cruel twist of fate for me to get type 1 diabetes, but it could have been a lot worse. I could have acquired a condition for which there was nothing I could do to alter the course of the disease. The truth is, I'm in a perfect position to deal with type 1 diabetes. I'm a highly disciplined individual by nature. I'm a physician with a firm understanding of human physiology, and I have medical knowledge of the importance of maintaining blood glucose in a normal range. Working in an academic medical center, I have access to people like my nurse practitioner, and I am fortunate in having the financial resources to obtain whatever care I need."

David views his diabetes purely as the need for hormone replacement therapy for insulin deficiency, similar to that of taking thyroid hormone for hypothyroidism. He has relegated the cumbersome details of providing insulin replacement to a "nuisance problem" like flossing his teeth. "It's a pain in the ass, but not a disease that will shorten my life. I accept it and feel resigned that I'm stuck with this, possibly for the rest of my life." When asked why he used the word "possibly," he states that he hopes there will be a cure for diabetes within ten years:

> I'm just trying to preserve the health of the endothelium [inner linings] of my blood vessels until then. In the short term, there will be an automatic system for my insulin pump, so I won't have to make decisions every hour about my blood sugar and insulin needs. The pump will be programmed to make adjustments automatically, based on my blood sugar. In the long term, I hold hope that a cure will come from stem cells that can turn off the disorder which destroys the insulin-secreting cells in my pancreas.[2]

After five years, David no longer feels that diabetes is a death sentence. He believes, with his ability to control diabetes tightly, he should not suffer any of the serious complications that can affect people with diabetes. "It is important for my self-concept not to view type 1 diabetes as a disease, and I refuse to view myself as sick. I still consider myself to be in excellent health, even though it takes a lot more work to maintain my health than it used to. Even with diabetes, I'm healthier than most people I know."

The account of this patient is not intended to exemplify the average or usual personal approach to the presence of diabetes. It does represent the most vigorous and self-disciplined response we have encountered.

CHAPTER 6

E-mails from Angela

January 2003

Dear Kathleen,

I am enclosing my blood sugar reports for the past few days. The only low one was when I forgot to decrease my insulin dose like you told me.

I went to a diabetes seminar at a local hospital tonight. I was the youngest person there by a solid twenty years. I don't think most people in that room had a clue about my type of diabetes. I have come to the conclusion that instead of "type 1" and "type 2" they need to come up with completely different names for these two conditions, because I really don't think I have the same disease as those people. The doctor who gave the lecture recommended testing the blood sugar twice a week. I test more than that every day. Did you know that they don't even have an endocrinologist on staff at that hospital. The nurse told me they're getting one in a few months. She also told me that just last week someone came in to the ER with an insulin pump, and they freaked out. They didn't know what to do with him. I am planning a trip to the tattoo studio right now—"DO NOT TAKE ME TO THAT HOSPITAL" will be permanently written on my skin. One lady at the seminar thought that if she ignored diabetes, it might just go away. If I ignored her, would she go away?

And for the last subject, anniversaries. My one-year diabetes anniversary is coming up next Sunday. I'm trying to decide how best to mark the event. I thought about doing it like they do in Alcoholics Anonymous (since someone I met during the last year compared having diabetes to alcoholism) and having my one-year cake. But I guess that would be like an alcoholic having a keg to commemorate. I shot down that idea. I told my husband that I could stop taking my shots and re-create the episode of DKA, but he said "No," then he said, "Hell, No." So that idea was canned. I have to work that day, so the anniversary celebration may be minimal. If you have any suggestions, let me know. Otherwise, I'll just wake up in my bed and not on the bathroom floor after throwing up and having dry heaves all night. I'll go to church and pray for the quacks at the walk-in clinic who missed the diagnosis of DKA. I'll go to work and not to the emergency room. I'll breathe in and out slowly all day and not hyperventilate. I'll braid my hair as the ICU nurse did, after she cleaned me up, to help me remember how little things can make all the difference. I'll call home and apologize again for putting them through all that. I'll be extra nice to my husband, who had the "in sickness" part tested after just barely a year of marriage.

And I'll do my shots, because this is now my life.

Thanks for listening.
Angela

Sometime in 2004
Dear Kathleen,
Many new and strange words are thrown at a person when first diagnosed with diabetes. I remember the first time I heard "DKA" or even Diabetes, for that matter. I was lying on an exam table in the emergency department of the very same Florida hospital where I had been brought into the world twenty-five years earlier. It was a Saturday afternoon in January of which I can only remember bits and pieces. I remember hearing those letters being uttered by the doctor and wondering what this abbreviation stood for. I could, however, already tell you what they meant to me: the hyperventilation, the nausea and vomiting, the headache, the muscle pain was nothing compared to the fear of not knowing what was happening to me and the uncertainty of knowing whether this person could do anything to make it stop.

I had once heard my high school French teacher say that in order to learn a new language, it is best to be totally immersed in the culture speaking that language. Over the next few days, I became fluent in Diabetes, even learning the true definition of DKA. I have to honestly say I didn't fight learning this new language. I realized that this was the only way to keep this awful nightmare from returning. I was immersed. Carbs were no longer something related to the latest diet fad. I learned the meaning of a sliding scale and that syringes are not needles. I learned what a lancet is (a word I still don't like) and about the world of blood glucose meters. But there are two words that I feel are always going to be in a state of flux: Control and Compliant. Am I in Control? Am I Compliant?

When I talk about Control, I am not just speaking of an A1c reading under 7 percent. Control comes in many forms and my level of Control oscillates from day to day. Yes, it does refer to blood glucose, but it can also stand for getting through a day without being surprised by this disease. No unexpected highs or unexplained lows. When I make it a week without catching my pump on my office desk, I call that Control. I have even started to define it as not being a smart-aleck to the ignorant members of society when I hear the sentence, "Should you be eating that?" I feel not throwing the nearest office supply at these people shows amazing Control. I have had these well-meaning do-gooders even remind me that desserts have sugar in the ingredients at my company Christmas party. Control is not a box that can be checked either "Yes" or "No," because in reality it changes from day to day, hour to hour, moment to moment. This disease does not want to be Controlled and it will fight you every step of the way to gain that Control.

Compliance can be just as vague. It can vary as much as the weather. I find myself eating a healthy lunch and following it up with a trip to Ben and Jerry's. Does this make me compliant with my diagnosis? Images in society can put Compliance on the back burner. I like watching game shows as I huff and puff away on my treadmill. Recently, the prize for the contestant on a game show I had tuned in to was a treadmill, and the model showing it off was a leggy beauty walking on it wearing an evening gown and high heels. That really made me feel like jumping off, but I stayed on and the Compliance pendulum swung a little higher. That was a Tuesday. I can't say I would have done the same on Wednesday.

Shortly after my hospitalization, I was at a greeting card store buying thank you notes for the many family and friends who came to my aid during this crazy time. One card caught my eye and I ended up buying it but never sending it out. It was a card for me. It remains in a frame on my desk to this day. On the front was a little girl with a frustrated expression leaning over a bowl of food. Over the top of the photo was a quote attributed to Anton Chekhov: "Any idiot can face a crisis, it's this day-to-day living that wears you out." That sums up what I feel continues to be a theme in my Diabetic Life, so all I can do is try to keep the pendulum swinging high and keep buying myself greeting cards.

Angela

Sometime in 2005
Dear Kathleen,
I have started this test this morning, and it has already brought up a question. When I mark down the carbs counted . . . What if I guess wrong? What if one unit per eight grams is correct for my morning bolus, but I think I have eaten fifty grams when I really took in sixty-five? Do you want me to eat packaged foods that tell me the exact number of carbs? Or am I jumping ahead of the game? Or are you alarmed that I am asking this, since I should be better at this by now? I have been dealing with this since January of 2002; shouldn't I know what I'm doing by now?

I was thinking this morning about my first few meals after "the big day." Can you imagine that I remember them? I have no idea what I ate, but I think back to being in the hospital and giving myself a shot and waiting for the onset. I was so scared to eat before the thirty minutes was up, because I thought I might go into DKA again. I think back and laugh. What a complete moron I was at the time!

Remember when pumps were so huge . . . they were the size of pagers!

Remember when insulin had to be refrigerated!

Remember when we used to have to stick ourselves with a needle every time we needed to test!

Remember when diabetes was cured, and we all burned our pumps and meters and syringes and lancets and said Goodbye Forever!!

Well, on to the future!

Angela

Spring 2006
Dear Kathleen,
Do you think we could fix my pump so that in addition to insulin, I could bolus Valium when I have to deal with stupid people? What do you think?

I hope you had a good vacation. I had a few little mishaps while you were out, but Anne took good care of me.

I recently purchased a "new-to-me" car. I was very excited to get this car and proceeded to read the owner's manual cover to cover. (I never needed to do this with my old car, since it had no special electronic features, and the only maintenance I ever had to do was feed the hamster who ran on the wheel that powered the engine). As I was reading, I came across the fuel portion. How to fill up your gas tank 101 . . . hmmm . . . I wondered . . . what could I really learn from this? It is not surprising that I didn't learn much about fuel, but it is shocking what I learned about Diabetes.

The recommendation about filling up a gas tank is this: Fill up at the same gas station using the same pump with the car facing the same direction *every* time. What!? Same gas station? In these days of nearly $3 a gallon gasoline, the cheapest station wins out. Most times cars are filled at whichever station is convenient. Same pump? Maybe by coincidence, if no one else is using it already. Car facing the same direction? As long as I'm not being blinded by the sun, I face a direction so that the gas tank of my car is on the side closest to the pump. Does anyone really do this? Is anyone able to plan their life out to be so predictable that they know that the car will run out of gas at the very moment they pass by the one gas station they are permitted to use, wait for the correct pump, and turn the car around to face the same direction?

No one would really think of doing this. It seems ridiculous. So why, then, am I asked by friends, why I can't just eat the same thing every day at the same time every day to control my blood sugar? And this seems logical to them?

The simple answer is this: Just as in my car, the route I take changes, the traffic flow varies, and gas prices rise and fall. In my daily routine the food I eat, the exercise I do, the stress I have changes all the time. It is never as simple as "eat the same thing every day." Besides, who wants to do that? Imagine trying to decide what breakfast you will eat for the rest of your life. Blueberry pancakes or mushroom omelets? Waffles with maple syrup or cereal with fruit? Ok

... so maybe I could eat blueberry pancakes every day for the rest of my life, but what happens when I go out to eat and blueberry pancakes aren't on the menu?

Variety is indeed the spice of life. If I had to fill up my car at the same station each time, using the same pump, facing the same direction, I could never leave the area. I could never go on a road trip with my friends, visit my family, see the country, and experience the wonder that discovery brings. If I had to eat the same thing every day, I couldn't have cake on my birthday, buttery popcorn at the movies, or even just try a new recipe in my own kitchen.

No . . . that definitely is not for me. I think I will take my chances filling up whenever and wherever and do my best to stay in control along the way.

Angela

May 2007
Dear Kathleen,
I love roller coasters. Love. L-O-V-E roller coasters. At any amusement park, I am always on the lookout for these rumbling giants with their twisted steel glimmering in the sun. They are my idea of the perfect ride, the ultimate combination of mouthwatering anticipation and adrenaline pumping, hands in the air, wind in my hair, feet dangling, screaming fun. When I was in high school, my Physics teacher took us to Busch Gardens to study the properties of the roller coasters (I always loved Physics). Even the school newspaper that I photographed for got in the game and did a big story when the park unveiled the newest gem in their coaster crown. Best of all, I never get sick riding. I was actually on several roller coasters the day before I was diagnosed with diabetes. I felt a little queasy and thought this was the beginning of symptoms of inheriting my parents' motion sickness, which so far had joyfully skipped my gene pool. Once I found out that those symptoms were that of DKA and not some evil dormant motion sickness gene, there was a small part of me that was relieved that I was still going to be able to ride.

What I didn't realize at that time was that I was unwittingly already on a roller coaster. Mouthwatering is replaced with a dry, parched mouth and a thirst that an ocean couldn't quench. I now

pump insulin, not adrenaline. The wind that danced through my
fingertips when my hands were high above my windblown hair are
now routinely pricked. I am constantly warned about what might
happen to my feet.

I hate diabetes. Hate. H-A-T-E diabetes. I hate the highs and
lows that seem like they can happen at the speed of those coasters.
I despise meter reading that can send my head spinning faster than
a 120' tall wraparound corkscrew. The looks of disapproval when
having dessert are equal to those I imagine a pregnant woman would
get when in line for some of these rides. Everyone else always knows
better and the murmurs I hear are as loud as laying an ear to the track
might be.

And then I try to scream. I try to tell someone to stop this ride.
I yell that I am tired of it. I scream to let me off, but no one is able to
help me. I yell and scream so much I leave myself mute. No one can
hear me now. I just keep going and going on this untamed monster,
spinning, jolting, diving, soaring forever. There is no station to get off.
No brakes to stop it. Now I am sick. I imagine unbuckling myself and
letting momentum have its way; it already seems like it is anyway. But
I can't get the latch undone and just end up with vomit all over me.

Some roller coasters have places in the track that will slow a car
down if it has too much momentum going into the next segment. I
search for that, long for it. I need it.

I can't imagine being on this ride forever.

Angela

Spring 2008
Dear Kathleen,
If I had a day off . . .

In January, I returned to the university where I received my
Bachelor's degree 9 years ago, to study for a Master's degree. I was
walking to class at dusk along the "old" part of campus (where no
new buildings had been erected), when suddenly, the years since
graduation disappeared. I was 20 years old and had woken from a
dream that was all the years I have lived since then. It only lasted
a moment, but in that moment, so much of my current reality was
gone, including diabetes. I was a co-ed, not the pincushion I am

today. I juggled books and classes and assignments. I saw my future being rosy, not covered in droplets of blood. And I danced on my toes without a second thought. And this tiny hitch in time made me think . . . what if I could be that carefree again, just for a day . . .

If I had a day off from diabetes, I would wake up wearing a nightgown since it wouldn't matter that my pump had no place to clip on. If I had a day off from diabetes, my morning would not start off by seeing blood (no matter how small the drop needs to be) and having a little computer tell me how I am doing. I would decide how I'm doing. If I had a day off from diabetes, I would take a shower and not want to wash away all the marks on my belly. If I had a day off from diabetes, I might take a morning vitamin to keep myself healthy, but then again, I might not. If I had a day off from diabetes, I would wear a dress to the park and walk barefoot through the grass. And I wouldn't carry a purse filled with all the things I might need "just in case." If I had a day off from diabetes, I would go swimming and not worry about the "pump button" [infusion set] showing through my bathing suit. Getting a tan would be my biggest concern. If I had a day off from diabetes, losing the 100 grams my pump weighs would make me feel 100 pounds lighter.

On my day off, the TV remote would be the only thing I would have to control. My calendar would be clear of doctor's appointments and full of gatherings with friends. My medicine cabinet would only contain toothpaste and my wallet would be a lot thicker. On my day off, I wouldn't have to explain to anyone what I am doing or that my pump is not a pager. And on my day off, I would think about the company I keep and not the disease that follows me around. On my day off, I would dance on my toes.

I had 9,148 days without diabetes. Did I squander those days? Did I appreciate what I had when I had it? Why now does diabetes leak into my memories? Sometimes I think, "How did I check my blood sugar in high school?" and then I remember that I didn't have diabetes then. Every day it robs me of my most intimate moments, why then must it rob me of my past too?

I want it to be over. I want to have that moment where I wake up and realize it has all been a dream, just like that moment on campus.

Somebody wake me up . . . please.

Angela

CHAPTER 7

A Difficult Decision

Dianne had type 1 diabetes that had never really been in adequate control. She admitted difficulty in remembering to take insulin injections at meals, in counting carbohydrates, and in just finding the time to attend to the daily details of diabetes care. Anne and I had started seeing Dianne as a team when she was eighteen, after she had graduated from high school. She was able to make some small improvements, but she often missed appointments and couldn't make diabetes enough of a priority in her life.

Anne recalls, "I was aware that Dianne had a boyfriend, and on more than one occasion, we had discussed the risk of pregnancy. She was counseled repeatedly about the ineffectiveness of her contraceptive practices, about the importance of planning for pregnancy, and about the necessity of optimal control of diabetes before pregnancy." Since the baby's organs form during the first few weeks of pregnancy, even before the first missed menstruation, the presence of high blood sugar then can cause serious birth defects in the fetus.

The phone call came to Anne: a home pregnancy test had been positive. Anne told Dianne to come to the clinic immediately. It had been six weeks since her last menstrual period and four weeks since fertilization of the egg. Most of the major organ systems of the fetus had been initiated and were developing, either normally or abnormally. Anne arranged for Dianne to see me at once, as well as locating a demo insulin pump and enough supplies to start her on the pump later that afternoon.

Dianne's two most important laboratory tests were in her hand: the positive confirmation of her home pregnancy test, and the A1c test, which indicated that her average blood sugar for the preceding three months was about 300 mg/dl (normal is less than 100 mg/dl). "I never thought this would happen to me," she lamented.

With this level of blood sugar during the first six to eight weeks of pregnancy, the risk of a major congenital malformation is as high as 30 percent. Major congenital malformations are defined as abnormalities that are fatal to the newborn, require surgical correction, or lead to marked physical or mental handicaps. In the infant of a mother with diabetes, they most commonly affect the cardiovascular system or the central nervous system.

Several studies have indicated that the incidence of major congenital malformations is much lower in the offspring of women who participated in careful pre-pregnancy management of diabetes, and of women with planned pregnancies.

They were a well-dressed, serious, worried couple. Dianne said little. The father asked most of the questions, but they both already knew the answers. "What are the odds of losing the baby?" "What's the chance of having an abnormal baby?" "What if she starts getting the diabetes under control now?" Then the question I had known was coming: "Doctor, do you recommend an abortion?"

I pointed out that I had seen several women with blood sugars as high or higher during the first trimester who had gone on to have normal pregnancies and had delivered perfectly healthy babies. In fact, that was the case in two out of three. In my mind, the decision was going to depend on what level of risk this couple could accept.

The prospective parents remained in the clinic for three hours. Anne taught Dianne how to use an insulin pump, and Dianne agreed to start testing her blood sugar at least four times each day—never a priority for her before that afternoon. It seemed the world had changed suddenly. As Dianne and her boyfriend left the clinic, their last words were, "We've got to make a very difficult decision."

Dianne decided to proceed with the pregnancy. Over the next few days, she returned to the clinic frequently until she was capable of using the insulin pump appropriately. We arranged for her to attend the High Risk Obstetrics Clinic. During pregnancy, she gained sixty-four pounds and had high blood pressure and swelling up to the knees (preeclampsia). Her infant was delivered by cesarean section because of its large size. Born with a congenital heart abnormality that required surgery a year later, Dianne's daughter is otherwise healthy.

An older doctor once said, "I just tell all my girls with diabetes they can't get pregnant." In the past, pregnancies in women with diabetes did lead to excessive rates of complications, including miscarriages, birth defects, stillbirths, serious medical problems in newborn infants, and/or severe illness or even death of the mothers. However, modern treatment makes it feasible to maintain near-normal blood sugar levels both before conception and during pregnancy. These days, the rates of these complications in women with diabetes are just slightly above those in women without diabetes, and healthy pregnancies can be expected. The key is pre-pregnancy planning, which should begin in adolescence. Unfortunately, unplanned pregnancies occur in more than half of women with diabetes, as it did in Dianne.

Alc levels should be as close to normal as possible before conception is attempted. The goals for blood sugar should be between 80 mg/dl and 110 mg/dl before meals and below 155 mg/dl two hours after meals. Once the patient has achieved blood sugar control that is as stable as she can achieve, then contraception can be discontinued.[1] During pregnancy, the goals will be even lower.

CHAPTER 8

A Life without Control

Sickness doesn't travel in straight lines.
—Rita Charon[1]

Clint had been incarcerated for the previous twenty-five years. When I met with him, he had been released from prison three months before. He was living with his mother and other family members, and he said he couldn't get a job. At the time of his discharge from prison, his weight had been normal, but now his diabetes was terribly out of control, and he had lost twenty pounds. He looked emaciated, as though he had been in a concentration camp.

I couldn't understand why his diabetes had been controlled better in prison than at home. He explained to me:

> When I was inside prison, I felt comfortable with diabetes. My blood sugar was usually between 180–250 mg/dl. I felt good. My weight was normal. In prison, I went to the clinic the first thing every morning, they stuck my finger. I'd get a shot twice a day: they would watch me give the shot, then I'd give the needle back.
>
> Next I went to the cafeteria, but I went through a special diet line. I would get one piece of toast, egg whites, and a piece of bacon that I could almost see. I think it was 2,200 calories. There were no choices—they would put the food on the tray. The food was good. Some of the other guys who didn't have diabetes wanted my food instead of theirs. I didn't have to wait in a long line, I'd be out and gone back to my unit before they were through eating. To make sure you stuck to your diet, if you didn't get your tray they would charge you $1 for each

meal. That made me get three meals each day, I didn't want to pay $3.

At lunchtime, if my number was high, I'd get another shot. If my blood sugar was real high, they'd put me in a little cell by myself with a pitcher of cold water. I would stay there until I drank the whole pitcher of water to bring it down.

They had me on a controlled diet, but once I got out, there was no such thing as a controlled diet. Inside, I knew what I had to do. I exercised, I ran track, lifted weights, played basketball if I could run, tried to play baseball if my leg wasn't tight. When we couldn't go out, I would walk around the unit. All the way around it twenty times was a mile; I would do 100 laps.

When asked what had changed since he was released from prison, Clint replied, "It's not how my diabetes is doing, it's how I'm doing." Clint described his current situation:

It's more stressful for me being out than it was on the inside. I get kinda lazy myself, about not doing everything that needs to be done. I forget to take my shot sometimes, don't check my sugar, stuff like that. If I feel bad and go to sleep, I just wait until the morning to take my shot. I get thirsty when I miss a shot. Sometimes I have a problem getting strips for two or three weeks. I don't have no money.

I stay with Momma and them. There's just too much going on there, I need my own place. I tore a piece of skin on my foot, it got infected, and my leg had to be amputated. Now nobody wants to mess with me. I give my own insulin shots, but nobody helps me put on my clothes, they don't have time. When I was locked up, I could get someone to help me. Now, maybe I can bribe my little nephew, give him $2 to help me occasionally.

I asked Clint about how he'd grown up. "The area was strictly ghetto," he recounted. "I've been where it's poor, and wondering where the next meal was coming from. There were eight boys, I was the oldest one at home. The oldest took care of the next one, the next one took care of the next one, and down the line. When I was twelve, I had a paper route, I'd take my money and buy clothes for my brothers, stuff like that. I didn't know my father until I was fourteen. I met him shooting dice, he took my money. I ran home and told my momma that some man took my money. I looked out the door, and that man was sitting in front of the house. My momma said, 'That man is your daddy.'"

Clint reminisced, "When I was twelve, I could throw a ball three hundred feet, from deep center field to home plate. I was good enough to play professional baseball, but I messed up my knee." Clint had won a track scholarship to a junior college in Tennessee, but didn't run track there. Instead, as a walk-on, he played point guard on the basketball team for two years.

Clint related that his first conviction was for homicide, at age twenty-three. Subsequently he received at least three more sentences, including nine-year and eleven-year prison terms for selling drugs. "Some of my best friends from high school are lawyers, schoolteachers, and dentists. I know how to do the right thing. I had a chance to do right, but I messed up. I don't hold anyone else responsible for any of that—it's all on me."

He was diagnosed with diabetes when he was thirty-nine, sixteen years ago. Diabetes is also present in his grandmother, mother, and at least one brother. Clint described his feelings at the onset of diabetes: "At first I said, it ain't nothing, I feel good, I ain't going to worry about nothing." He lamented, "If I had started taking care of myself then, this may not have happened. I need to turn myself around. I'm not helping myself by being lazy. Diabetes will take me away whenever the good Lord wants to take me away."

But then his swagger reappeared. "The only thing that helped me was being an athlete, you know what I mean? Guys come up to me now and say, 'You still shoot ball?' I ain't shot no ball for twenty years. But that's what they knew me as. I was the smallest man on the court, but I was as good as any of them. No one could say he was better than me. Some of them would say they'd rather play against a five-man team than play me one-on-one."

Regarding the role of medical care in his life, Clint said, "When I go to doctors, they always say the same thing. I already know what they'll say. 'You're doing OK, we'll see you again in three months.' Some may ask how you feel, or how you're doing, but my experience is, once you start telling them about your life or your problems, they go blank."

As a young man, Clint had been a heroin user and he had shared needles. He acquired HIV and hepatitis A, B, and C. Now the HIV is under control with four potent drugs, and his liver function tests are virtually normal. It is diabetes that is destroying his health. He has the classic symptoms of uncontrolled diabetes—unquenchable thirst and passing urine every few hours. He eats all the food his mother cooks for him, but it seems to pass right through him. His muscles are melting away.

CHAPTER 9

We Control What We Can

Kathleen first met Otto in the spring of 2002. She recalls,

Otto appeared robust, fit, and younger than expected for his sixty-nine years. He had some strong opinions about his diabetes and clearly didn't plan to take my word blindly. I asked him to keep records of his blood sugar and fax them to me. This request must have struck him as being sensible, because he began sending me records every week, and, to my surprise, he has continued this practice for over five years now. These log sheets often contain a personal message related to his blood sugar level. At some point he began adding another statement, which he called a "cliché," at the bottom. On July 24, 2006, I found this handwritten note at the bottom of his weekly blood sugar report: "Kathleen, after my 7-day stay at the V[eterans] A[dministration] Hospital, all the results of testing and biopsies are in. I have received results that I have cancer of the kidney. It is not curable. I'm glad I'm back to managing my blood sugar—the VA sure couldn't manage it."

Otto's cancer had spread to the lymph nodes and the lungs. His doctors had indicated that his life expectancy was less than eighteen months. Two different types of chemotherapy had caused severe side effects and had shown no benefit whatsoever.

A week later, Otto faxed a blood glucose record with the following words at the bottom of the page: "As you can see, I have got hold of my sugar. I always said, it's all in the diet. Thought for the day: 'I asked for all things, that I might enjoy life. I was given life, that I might enjoy all things.'"[1]

The next week, Otto's blood sugar record had these words at the bottom of the page: "Kathleen, because I am deathly sick 24/7 from cancer medication and I can't eat normally, I have lost control of my sugar, as my numbers reflect. Now my blood sugar is too low. I have been using sugar in milk as a quick fix, however that lasts only for an hour or so."

Expecting that diabetes had become second fiddle, clinically outranked by his cancer, I drove out to Otto's home, located about an hour west of Nashville. "We like it here," he said. "I retired and bought this mobile home. It's all my wife and I need. My son lives down the road, and my daughter lives three miles away. This is where it'll all end, right here. I'm on borrowed time now. There's no cure, no medication."

Otto described the area around his home: "They raise tobacco, corn, and hay here, alternating those crops. Most people work in Nashville and farm as a sideline. You have to be careful driving at night around here, because deer are so numerous. This season of the year, the bucks are growing their horns, and the does have their little fawns. Later on, those bucks will be chasing those does everywhere."

Before discussing his medical condition, we reviewed Otto's life. "My father played harmonica and drums," he said. "From the time I was a child in New York City, I was a musician. I played drums for twenty-five years, and a little harmonica, but now I play harmonica all the time. I also was in the collision repair business and owned body shops all over the United States. The day job was kinda secondary to me. Playing music, that was my forte."

Six years ago, his daughter heard of a harmonica teacher at the Renaissance Center in nearby Dickson and decided to take lessons. Otto decided to go with her. "I went just to see how good the teacher was. He turned out to be a four-time national champion. My daughter quit after her five initial lessons, but I still go every Wednesday and take advanced training from him. My teacher is so impressed with the way I play, he wants me to make a CD. If there's enough time in my life, maybe I will."

Otto has a glass case on the wall displaying harmonicas he's worn out. "The reeds bend, and a note could become sharp or flat. I usually play a harmonica called a sextet. It has six different harmonicas on it, each with a different key. Every Monday, I play at a restaurant where my daughter is the chef. I play easy listening music, and people respond well. They say they've never seen no harmonica like that. Every time I play harmonica, I play a patriotic tribute. And God bless the VA, because they're treating my cancer. That's one of the most wonderful organizations. That bottle of pills would have cost $6500 if I had to buy it."

When I asked Otto about his current health, he replied, "As far as diabetes goes, I have a handle on it. The first thing in the morning, I check my sugar and have a cup of coffee. If my blood sugar is high, I put Splenda in it. If it's low, I put sugar in it."

I asked Otto's wife what she thought about his taking better care of his diabetes now that he had another problem that was more serious. "He's done absolutely wonderful since he has been watching his diet," she answered. "He had always watched it some, but he does it more so now. That sugar thing is very scary."

I asked Otto how the treatment for the tumor had dominated the treatment for diabetes. "It hasn't dominated it," he said. "It has had some effect. My blood sugar seems more erratic when I take the chemo pills. Before this cancer business, I wasn't taking as much precaution with what I was eating, and my sugar was up and down. Now I try to do as much as I can to control the diabetes. I eat better. I don't want to carry the excess weight. The 240 pounds was too much for me. It had a bad effect on the diabetes. Now that I'm down to 208, I feel better, and it reflects on my blood sugar readings."

I was astonished at this answer. I had assumed that focusing on the more imminent problem of cancer would have diminished his attention to self-care of diabetes. "Why do you take better control of the diabetes now that you have cancer?"

"Well, I don't know exactly," he replied. "I'm whipping a dead horse. Now that I'm dying, I'm starting to take better care of myself. I'm trying to stay here as long as I can for my children and my wife. I know that's like closing the door of the barn after the horse gets out. My harmonica instructor says, 'You just keep on playing,' and I agree with him."

Patients with diabetes are living longer, increasing their chance of acquiring one of the many chronic diseases associated with aging. Some coexisting conditions are so complex or serious that they eclipse the management of diabetes.[2] Terminal cancer would be one such example, I had presumed.

There are some things in life over which we have no control. But rather than forfeit all control, we control what we can.

CHAPTER 10

The Cadillac of Disabilities

The voice processor on Arlene's cash register speaks like an automaton: "Three point six three is your change." She claims it never makes a mistake unless she pushes the wrong button.

Arlene lost her vision as a result of diabetic retinopathy at age twenty-six, but now, at age fifty-one, she is self-sufficient. I spent a day watching her operate a snack counter and service her vending machines at the State Capitol in Nashville. "I hope I'm not in food service for the rest of my life," she said, "but it pays my bills now."

I noticed that she always kept her finger on the number five key on her cash register. "The five always has a little bump on it—on cash registers, calculators, and phones," she enlightened me. I grabbed for my cell phone. Sure enough, there was a little bump I had never noticed on the number five key.

The snack counter was busy with a steady string of customers—legislators, lobbyists, members of the press, and visitors. "I can spot the newsmen," she joked. "Sometimes they act like they just woke up."

Customers constantly walked behind her, getting food or drinks out of the refrigerator or freezer cases. "I made it self-serve. I couldn't take care of people asking me to get a sandwich and get a coke while I was trying to work the cash register too," she explained. "I have many types of sandwiches. Most have to be warmed in the microwave behind me here." Microwave popcorn, fresh fruit, candy, snack crackers, muffins, pastries, doughnuts, soft drinks, bottled tea and cappuccino, ice cream, yogurt, tacos, chimichangas, and chicken wings are just a few of the items on her shelves.

"The governor's favorite coffee is Starbucks, so that's what I sell, and I sell a lot of bottled water. I'm fortunate because the old water fountains in the capitol building don't work well," she said. "Candy is my biggest seller—really ironic for someone who has diabetes and has a master's degree in health education."

In the vending machines on the floor below, she sells frozen dinners also. Her bill-changing machines are programmed to spit out quarters only. "If someone changes a $20 bill, they get eighty quarters. I don't know what they do with that many quarters, unless they need to do their laundry."

Arlene was a dental hygienist before she lost her vision:

I first noticed floaters, followed by a big vitreous hemorrhage in my right eye. Then I had a smaller hemorrhage in my good eye. I had surgery on my good eye—a vitrectomy—to prevent it from doing what the right eye had done. The operation failed, and I totally lost my sight in my left eye. Then I developed glaucoma in it. I lost my vision and my job. There isn't much demand for a dental hygienist who can't tell if the mouth is open.

When I first lost my sight, I asked the ophthalmologist, "What do I do now? I'm a dental hygienist and I teach calligraphy. Everything I do is visual." He replied, "You're just going to have to learn to be blind."

Since then, I've had three vitrectomies on my right eye. I'm thankful for just a little bit of sight there. My visual acuity is about 20/600. [20/600 means that Arlene's vision is reduced to the point that she must be at twenty feet to see what she should normally be able to see at six hundred feet. 20/200 is considered legally blind.]

Contacts help trim up the blurs a little bit. I use these magnifying glasses for things like eating. I can see people are there. If it's real bright or contrasted, I may be able to tell what they're wearing. I can see a little of your face now, your hair is grayish.

I can see the numbers on my glucose meter, because they are very contrasted. The display on the glucose meter is black on a light grey, better than most. White on black would be great, it jumps out at you better. I wish the meter manufacturers would think about the problems of visually impaired people. Also, I don't understand why they haven't developed an insulin pump for us.

When I lost my sight after the operation, I was depressed. I stayed with my parents for two months. Some people who had known me all my life wouldn't come up and talk to me. They acted like they didn't know I was the same person. I was dating someone when I lost my vision. He dropped me like a hot potato, and that was hurtful. I wasn't married, and I thought, "Who would want to marry a blind girl?"

My parents were very sheltering. I remember just sitting and rocking in their den, because I didn't have anything else to do. Then I decided to move back to my apartment in Murfreesboro. I did spring cleaning; I just had to try and see what I could do. The more I tried, the more I found I could do. The hardest thing to give up was driving. Sometimes I would just move my car up and back four feet in the driveway. One day the phone rang and an excited neighbor said, "You've got your sight back! I saw you moving your car in the driveway."

Taking care of my apartment started me back on the road to healing. Then I learned about a special camp for the blind in South Carolina where they had horseback riding, archery, sailing, canoeing, and water skiing. I had tried water skiing many times in the past. I could never get up. When I tried to ski at the camp, I got up the first time. I guess it was because I wasn't looking at everything. When I learned that I could water ski, it made me think I could do other things.

I asked Arlene when she started dating again:

On my first date after I lost my sight, this fellow took me to a steak place for dinner. I was determined to be very independent and do everything myself. We got our steak and potato and I buttered the potato. I could put artificial sweetener in my iced tea; it seemed easy. It was a little dark in that place. At one point I cut off a huge bite of steak, and I had to open my mouth wide just to get this big piece in my mouth. I put my napkin over my mouth. Finally I chewed it all up and swallowed it. I looked at my date; I knew he wasn't going to say anything, so I started to cut another piece of steak, but there was no more. "What happened to the rest of my steak?" I asked, and he said, "You just ate it." That huge bite of steak was the whole thing.

Teaching activities of daily living at rehab for the blind in Nashville was my first paying job after I was blind. I went in as a teacher because I refused to go to rehab for myself. I wasn't going to let them pat me on the head like a puppy. I knew how to do all this stuff. I would try to do it at home the night before and then teach it the next day. It wasn't hard. I could cook, so I could teach them how to cook. I could teach people to sew on buttons with a special needle that you didn't have to thread. Some blind people use sewing machines, but I gave my sewing machine to my mother. At first I thought I wouldn't have to iron any more, but there are substitute ways to do everything. You have to take what you've got and go from there.

Blindness is the Cadillac of disabilities, because there's so much adaptive equipment available. I have a talking clock and talking scales. In cooking I can do just about anything I want. I have a knife with a little screw. Using it, I can cut perfect slices. I have a thing called "Say When": you put it on the side of a cup and it tells when the cup is almost full, but I don't need it any more.

I worked at rehab for the blind for a year and then went back to school and got my master's in health education. I was told by the dean that I couldn't get a job in health education because of my vision. I entered the program without his blessing, but I made all As and one B. I specialized in nutrition and fitness.

After I married, we moved to Washington, DC. I lived in Alexandria and worked in Washington. I traveled alone on the subway system. I used a cane. I worked part-time in public relations at the White House during the Reagan administration. It had nothing to do with health education; I just wanted to be in the know while I was in Washington. I also worked part-time in health education on a contract basis. At the Lighthouse for the Blind, I taught health-related courses, from stress management to pre-skiing conditioning.

I got into teaching aerobics as a result of my blindness. While participating in an aerobics class one night, a lady behind me said, "Everyone in front of you is doing what the instructor is doing, but all of us behind you are doing what you're doing." I decided it would be easier to lead than to follow, and I taught aerobics classes for fifteen years.

When Arlene moved back to Nashville, her kidneys failed, and she had a kidney transplant in 1989.

My older brother was my donor. We were a 100 percent match. He always says that he gave me his best kidney, and that his golf swing is worse since he's lopsided now. I tell him that I never did gross things like belching in public until I got his kidney.

After the kidney transplant, I was restless. I had divorced and was living alone. I began teaching aerobics at a family health center and also started working as a health education assistant at the Cumberland Science Children's Museum. I got to teach the kids everything: heart, muscles, and bones. I eventually became the director of health education there.

Transportation for blind and visually impaired people in Nashville is the pits. The Metro Transit Authority will pick you up at home, but you have to reserve it a day beforehand. If something goes overtime, you might not get a ride home. It's hard to ask people for rides; you feel like you're intruding on their time. You don't want people who see you coming to say, "Oh, no, she's going to ask me for a ride."

Arlene doesn't use Braille because she finds it too slow. She receives books on tape from the Library of Congress. Sometimes she can see better on television than naturally. Once the television screen revealed a man whom she knew and she realized for the first time that he had a mustache. She uses an electronic device called Visual Tech that magnifies and increases contrast in front of her computer. Even with this adaptation, trying to read on a computer is stressful and very slow. Arlene realized that she needed a job where she didn't have to look at a computer. She had interviewed for several jobs, but when she walked in with her cane, she realized she would have to convince her potential employer that she could do the work. "I remember seeing people with canes before I was blind. I would be sure to walk out of their way," she related. "People have preconceived notions like 'Bless your heart, I'm sure you would be good at this job if you could see.'"

Arlene frequently ate lunch with a blind friend who was running a small grill in a state office building under the auspices of Tennessee Business Enterprises (TBE). This federally funded program offers entrepreneurial opportunities in food services to visually impaired persons. "I had worked at a Dairy Queen at age sixteen, and I hated it. I said I never wanted to do anything in food again," Arlene recounted. "But TBE would help me get started, provide a training program, then provide vending machines or a food counter location. After that it would be mine to maintain and to work. I would be responsible for the business; it would be a private business. Many facilities across the state include food services at federal, state, and county buildings, state universities and colleges, even the profitable commissaries at the prisons."

Arlene's business includes the state capitol, the public library, and two other nearby buildings. At the capitol, just outside the chamber of the state legislature, she jokes with her customers. One of the legislators said, with a wink, "I'm putting my kids through college on Arlene. I always tell her I hand her a $50 bill, when it's really just a dollar bill, but she's on to me. She must have eyes in the back of her head."

Those who know Arlene tell her what items they have selected and slide the money into her hand. If the customer doesn't realize that she's blind, she just says, "Hi, what do you have? I can't see it, just tell me." She explained, "I have to put them at ease. Educating other people about blindness is one of the hardest things I do. People need to know that in diabetes, there is life after complications."

Diabetes, particularly diabetic retinopathy, is the leading cause of new cases of blindness in adults in the United States. Regular eye exams through dilated pupils, either by an eye professional or retinal photography, allows early detection of retinopathy at a stage before the patient has experienced any visual symptoms. If a vision-threatening condition is detected, panretinal laser photocoagulation may prevent blindness.

President Franklin D. Roosevelt signed the Randolph Sheppard Act into law on June 20, 1936. The landmark legislation gave states the right to set up business enterprise programs for persons who were legally blind and gave blind participants in the program priority in operating vending facilities in federal buildings. Since then, most states have passed legislation that extends the same priority to other government buildings. Today, many licensed blind managers successfully operate food service facilities in private sector buildings as well.

PART II

Control of Diabetes Is a Family Affair

Diabetes is a family disease. The "patient" is defined as the entire family. The family—not the individual with diabetes alone—is the focus of treatment.
　　—Joe Solowiejczyk[1]

The narratives in this section demonstrate that diabetes affects the whole family and that the family affects the control of diabetes. Both the tenderness and the conflicts that are part of family relationships have major effects on diabetes. Understanding the influence of illness on the family necessitates understanding the family itself, not just the illness.

The mother of a teenager with diabetes told me, "Her diabetes has caused me more stress, worry, and sadness than anything in my life. She became selfish and could use diabetes to manipulate others."

A child whose mother developed diabetes said, "I remember the day. I was six years old. All of a sudden, my mother was in the hospital. From then on, our lives changed. Everything was timed around diabetes, and our family was controlled by illness. Hospitals and doctors dominated our life. I thought she could die at any moment. I just wanted a normal life, for her to be well. I was the only one of my friends who had a sick parent. I would resent her, get angry, then feel guilty. You had to treat her with kid gloves."

A woman who has diabetes described having to choose between exercising and helping her son do his homework. Typically, she helps her son. "[My children's] needs come first, before mine. I think having children has made diabetes control harder to achieve, because I'm no longer number one."

On the other hand, several patients told us that they couldn't have survived diabetes without the support of their families. One said, "It would be so much harder if I didn't have the support I've had—not nagging, but support. I don't know how many of those frustrations I could handle."

CHAPTER 11

A Family Affair

*Telling stories of illness is the attempt . . . to give
a voice to an experience that medicine cannot
describe.*
    —Arthur W. Frank[1]

When Sheldon comes to my office for treatment of diabetes, I try to discuss his blood sugar levels and insulin doses, but Sheldon wants to talk about exploring caves. Spelunking is what captivates Sheldon, not diabetes control.

He likes to tell about the episode of high blood sugar on the day he rappelled into Hooper's Well, a ninety-foot pit. Sheldon was wearing an insulin pump, and he had inserted his insulin infusion needle into a site on his buttocks, where it would be out of the way.

Sheldon wore a harness known to cavers as a Knots rig, with a foot cam, a knee cam, and pulley. Wearing this harness, he could climb thirty meters in shortly over one minute. Basically, one just runs up the cord like a ladder. It is well-suited for use with an insulin pump, as there is space both for his pump and for some food in front of his abdomen, where it can be reached.

Before entering the pit, his blood sugar had been 150 mg/dl, an acceptably safe level just slightly above normal. He rappelled deep into the pit, then rapidly climbed back up and out. After the second descent, he felt peculiar, rechecked his blood sugar, and determined that it had risen to 300 mg/dl. He took a supplemental dose of insulin that should have decreased the blood sugar. After the fourth rappel into the chasm, his blood sugar had risen to 600 mg/dl, despite the vigorous physical activity that usually lowered his blood sugar. He took a second extra dose of insulin and rappelled into the pit a fifth time. When he emerged, he decided to check the insulin infusion site on his buttocks. Since a group was present, he had to sneak behind some bushes where he could lower his pants. He found to his surprise that the tip of the infusion needle had pulled out from his skin, and the insulin was just flowing into the space under the bandage.

"More often, my blood sugar gets too low on a caving trip," he says. "If I do a vertical cave and am going to spend hours there, I'll carry cokes, candy bars, and a sandwich, usually peanut butter with honey or molasses. Occasionally, I have gotten lost in a cave. You're not a caver if you don't get lost a few times. The worst time, I missed my turn and ran into a wall. It was about 5:30 in the afternoon, about time for bat flight, so I just sat there and ate a candy bar. When a bat sat on my shoulder, I followed him out and found my exit. It was dark."

Diabetes has interrupted more than caving, however. Sheldon had developed diabetes at eighteen months of age. In his early thirties, he developed proliferative diabetic retinopathy and had a vitreous hemorrhage in his right eye. A blood vessel ruptured into the eyeball, preventing light from reaching his retina, and he lost total vision in that eye. After a few months of limited activity—including no spelunking—the blood gradually settled, and his vision improved. A month later, a second hemorrhage occurred, decreasing his vision to 20/400.

This time Sheldon's vision did not improve, even after several months. He had a delicate ophthalmological procedure called a vitrectomy, in which the blood was sucked out from the center of his eye. His vision improved. Two years later, a hemorrhage occurred in the left eye with consequences similar to what had occurred in the right eye. Subsequently, a vitrectomy restored his vision in the left eye also.

At age thirty-four, Sheldon met Tonya, who was then a fifteen-year-old high school freshman. Tonya loved the outdoors. She had been to Girl Scout camp, where she had learned rappelling and rock climbing. Tonya recounts:

> One day when I got home from school, Sheldon was sitting in our living room talking to Momma. I didn't even have time to check my makeup. My mom didn't consider caving a date. That was the only way I could get out of the house, to go caving. Momma went into the caves with us for several years.
>
> It wasn't just Sheldon's personality, it was the environment he loved to be in, the adventurous part that attracted me to him. We had many cave dates. Once we decided to go caving

with two other guys, but they got grounded by their parents. Sheldon got stuck taking me alone. I remember standing on top of a pit 200 feet deep. Sheldon rappelled down to the bottom and yelled up at me that it was beautiful down there, that I had to come down. He would stand at the bottom and belay me, so if I lost control, he would stop me from crashing to the bottom. Finally I rappelled down. I will never regret it. It was the most beautiful pit I'd ever been in. I guess he decided he'd keep me.

The year before we got married, Momma's health wouldn't allow her to go caving any more. She finally allowed us to go to a caving convention alone for the weekend. It was under the assurance that there would be two tents and we would be on our best behavior.

Sheldon was thirty-eight and Tonya was nineteen when they married. He had had diabetes for thirty-six years and declining kidney function for about ten years. Shortly thereafter, he developed kidney failure.

"About a year after we were married, Sheldon started getting sick," recalls Tonya. "We started going to doctors more frequently. By the following year, he began peritoneal dialysis at home. It gave us the freedom to continue to take day trips rock climbing, but not quite as much cave exploring as we would have liked."

Peritoneal dialysis is a procedure that substitutes for kidney function. A small tube is surgically inserted into the abdomen. Through this tube, large amounts of fluid flow into the abdominal cavity. After an hour or so, this fluid contains some of the waste products normally removed by functioning kidneys. It is then drained out of the abdomen and back into the bottle. This process was repeated several times each night while Sheldon slept.

After several months, Sheldon received a kidney donated by his mother. The fact that his transplanted kidney was from a living, close relative decreased the risk of rejection. His transplanted kidney started producing urine while Sheldon was still on the operating table and functioned well for several years. In order to prevent his immune system from rejecting the kidney, he had to take strong immunosuppressive drugs.

"Sheldon's mother was almost a perfect match," Tonya recounts. "Even though she had had breast cancer ten years earlier, she was able to donate one of her kidneys, and in 2001 Sheldon got what he was waiting for. This was the greatest gift a son could ever ask for, and it has showed me what kind of mother I want to be for our child."

Kathleen recalls how Sheldon looked before his kidney transplant. "His complexion was gray, pale, and sallow, and hair very thin. I knew he was slipping when he told me he no longer had the energy to go into a cave. Then, within a short time following his transplant, as if by miraculous rebirth, his color returned, his hair looked healthy again, and he returned to his hyperenergetic self."

Sheldon and Tonya resumed spelunking together. Tonya had become an expert in all aspects of Sheldon's diabetes care, including the proper food, the details of insulin administration, and the recognition and treatment of his frequent episodes of low blood sugar. Within a few months of Sheldon's successful kidney transplant, Tonya became pregnant.

When their daughter Grace was three months old, she became ill. She cried a lot, vomited after eating, and couldn't gain weight. Tonya describes what happened: "We kept telling the doctors that something was wrong with Grace, but nobody believed us. We were told that babies didn't get diabetes until they were toddlers. We tried to explain that Sheldon got diabetes before he was a toddler. Finally they found that her blood sugar was 297 mg/dl, indicating the diagnosis of diabetes, and at age five months she was sent to Vanderbilt to begin insulin treatment."

Tonya quickly became skilled in administering the tiny doses of insulin that were required for the baby. Now she had two family members who needed insulin and her care. Before her first birthday, Grace was started on an insulin pump at the pediatric department of the Vanderbilt Diabetes Center. "The pump has made it much easier to care for her," Tonya states. "I test her blood sugar about every two hours during the day, then at midnight and 3 a.m. If she's sick, I wake up more often because of intuition. I have learned to function as a sleep-deprived mom who walks around with a diaper bag that is heavier than my toddler. Now she's three years old and literally a mini of her father, diabetes and all. But Grace is easier to care for than Sheldon; her body hasn't been beat up and abused by diabetes so much, and she has better control of diabetes. My biggest concern is that if Sheldon gets sicker, I'll have to explain it to Grace."

Since he was already committed to immunosuppressive treatment for the rest of his life, Sheldon had decided that if a pancreas became available for transplantation, it was worth a try in an attempt to cure his diabetes once and for all. In 2003, Sheldon received the pancreas transplant. The pancreas was obtained from a cadaver, the body of a deceased person who had been willing to donate his organs for transplantation. For a while, the insulin-producing cells in the pancreas transplant functioned well, producing sufficient insulin so that Sheldon was able to stop insulin injections for the first time in forty-one years.

"I think he tasted every sugar-sweetened beverage on the market and ate at least one of every candy bar on the planet. I remember the first time he ate cotton candy. I thought I would never get him off the ceiling from all the sugar," says Tonya.

But even with continued use of immunosuppressive drugs, Sheldon's immune system could recognize the transplanted pancreas obtained from a nonrelated donor as more dissimilar from him than the kidney obtained from his mother. After six months, his immune system rejected the transplanted pancreas, and he had to resume insulin treatment with his insulin pump.

Kathleen says, "When I talked to Sheldon and Tonya, I was very upset that Sheldon's transplanted pancreas had failed, but they were both upbeat about it. They said Sheldon had loved living without diabetes for six months, but that he had spent nearly his entire life with diabetes, and he knew perfectly well how to live with it. I think the worst part for him was physical. He became very ill during the rejection process, and it took a long time to recover from this."

Subsequently, Sheldon and Tonya started a window-washing business. Sheldon says, "There is no window that I can't get to." They have resumed spelunking. About solo caving, Sheldon says, "You're not supposed to go alone; the ideal is three people per trip. Many people won't go caving with me because they're afraid they'll have to deal with my diabetes, so sometimes I have to go alone." Tonya adds, "If his blood sugar has been OK, and his strength has been OK, and I know what cave he's going to, and if he's done that cave before, it's OK. But he has to give me a callout time—a time when he's back in the car. If I don't get that call, I know he's still in the cave."

Three-year-old Grace was honored in the local newspaper, the *Pulaski Citizen*, on April 18, 2006, as the Pulaski Citizen of the Week. She was credited with saving her daddy's life twice. The first time, her mother was at work, and Grace was at home with Sheldon, who seemed to have dozed off in a rocking chair. When Grace tried to get him to play with her, she couldn't awaken him. She raced up the two flights of stairs leading from her family's basement apartment to her grandparents' home. "Grandma, there's something wrong with Daddy, he needs a Coke," she shouted. On another occasion, Tonya had told Grace to wake up her daddy for breakfast. When Sheldon wouldn't open his eyes, Grace dashed into the kitchen and excitedly told her mother, "I've got to check Daddy's blood, it's low." Tonya followed her into the bedroom and watched in disbelief as Grace climbed onto the bed, correctly took a sample of blood from Sheldon's finger, and inserted the strip into the glucose meter. She couldn't read the numbers, but she waited for the number to display and then showed the meter to her mother. As Grace had predicted, her daddy's blood sugar was indeed low. She ran to the kitchen to get him some juice.

When the family visits Grace's pediatric endocrinologist at Vanderbilt every three months, Sheldon often drops in unannounced to see me or, more frequently, Kathleen. One day Sheldon, Tonya, and Grace were visiting Kathleen in her office. Sheldon was reviewing his blood sugar records, while Grace was squirming in Tonya's lap. Both Sheldon and Grace began to act bizarrely. Tonya knew intuitively that both were experiencing low blood sugar. "You'll have to take care of yourself this time, Sheldon, I've got to take care of the baby," she said. Tonya was correct. Sheldon was able to treat his hypoglycemic reaction himself, though she kept an eye on him.

When I learned that Grace was going into caves with Sheldon and Tonya, riding in a harness strapped to Sheldon's chest as they rappelled, I had to get a photo of them doing this together. On the appointed day, I met the three of them for breakfast at a restaurant in Pulaski. I watched as Tonya counted every grape that Grace ate, carefully computing the carbohydrate content to calculate the insulin dosage. Grace had a huge appetite; she consumed almost eighty grams of carbohydrates during that breakfast.

On the way to Miller's Cave, near Campbellsville, I asked when Grace had started caving. Tonya replied that the first time Grace went into a cave was before she was born; the couple hadn't known that Tonya was eight weeks pregnant at the time. Sheldon added, "Tonya wasn't herself that day. She has a knack for climbing and crawling, but she was sluggish and couldn't maneuver like she usually does."

At the cave, Sheldon, Tonya, and Grace donned their boots, rubber pants and coats, and lighted caving helmets. The photograph accomplished, I indicated that I would be going. "Doc, you really should

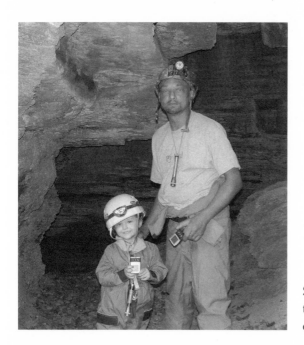

Sheldon and Grace with their insulin pumps at the entrance to Miller's Cave

see the first hundred feet of this cave," Sheldon contended. "There are beautiful mineral formations." After reluctantly crawling on my hands and knees through a muddy area, I acknowledged that the mineral formations were indeed picturesque.

Grace began to act fussy, but with the help of flashlights and the lights on the helmets, a quick check of her blood sugar revealed that it wasn't low as feared; a few minutes later, she was cheerful again. Her finger was pricked for blood sugar measurements eight times during the day I spent with them, a procedure she sometimes ignored if she was distracted.

Then Sheldon proposed that he explore another cavern alone—one requiring another long crawl—and that Tonya, Grace, and I wait for him in the high-ceilinged room near the cave entrance. "I'll join you in twenty minutes," he pledged.

While we waited, Tonya had time to reflect. "I won't say the last twelve years of my life have been hard, but I assure you it hasn't been normal. From marriage, to dialysis, to transplants, to having a child with diabetes. Who can say what normal really is? When I met Sheldon, I had no clue he was any different from anyone else. It took me a while, but I gradually realized he had a different routine from most people: he had diabetes. He took shots before meals and occasionally he needed an extra snack to bring up his blood sugar. I learned that even though he didn't look sick, he could become very sick very quickly if his blood sugar dropped too low."

As we sat in the dark cave, Tonya talked about the fact that Sheldon's transplanted kidney was failing. His name had been placed on the national transplant recipient list, and he was waiting for another kidney. Tonya related, "I was told not to give Sheldon one of my kidneys, because someday I might have to give it to Grace. This is killing me, because I'd like to help him. It's hard to make that decision; it's like watching a person drown and just standing on the dock and not helping."

After we had waited about an hour for Sheldon, I asked Tonya if she was concerned. "He knows this cave," Tonya replied. "He's probably not lost; he'll show up." Eventually he did, elated by the beauty of the mineral deposits he had seen. I was relieved that he was not unconscious from hypoglycemia. I had no injectable medical supplies with me, and without Sheldon, I would have been hopelessly lost in the cave.

CHAPTER 12

This Invisible Counterpart

*It is easier to change a man's religion
than to change his diet.*
—Margaret Mead

Peter is my son-in-law. I have known him since he was a freshman in college. From the beginning, I knew he loved four things: chips, salsa, chicken wings, and my daughter. His other favorites were pasta, french fried potatoes, and popcorn. Fun-loving and easygoing, he played basketball or soccer twice a week and coached in a youth soccer league. We all considered him healthy and fit. Since his high school days, he had noticed that he felt sluggish after eating sweets, so he never ate desserts. Instead, he prepared a huge bowl of popcorn in a hot-air popper after dinner every night and ate it all himself. We gave him a hard time about not offering to share his popcorn with the rest of the family, but apparently Peter justified his popcorn-hoarding by assuming that everyone else had already enjoyed their desserts.

Close scrutiny did disclose some concerns, however. Peter had insidiously gained about thirty pounds above his ideal body weight since high school. No one had noticed, since he was so active. At age thirty-seven, routine lab tests showed abnormalities in his lipid profile. His physician said that these lab results signified metabolic syndrome, which is present in about one-third of American adults. Peter's blood sugar was not then at a level to indicate diabetes, but his father, his paternal grandmother, and two of his great-uncles had developed diabetes in later years.

Peter was advised to lose weight. He was referred to a dietitian, and he shed seven pounds. Nevertheless, by the time of a life insurance exam two years later, measurements of his fasting blood sugar had shown a progressive increase from 120 to 125 to 135 mg/dl; a confirmed level above 125 mg/dl establishes the diagnosis of diabetes. Two hours after a meal, his blood sugar was 240 mg/dl; a level above 200 mg/dl is also diagnostic of diabetes. There was no question that, at the age of thirty-nine, Peter had diabetes.

Shortly thereafter, Peter's eleven-year-old niece developed type 1 diabetes. As a result, all of her close relatives, including Peter's three children, participated in TrialNet, an international network dedicated to the study, prevention, and early treatment of type 1 diabetes. Trial-Net searches for individuals at risk for future development of type 1 diabetes by screening for pancreatic islet cell antibodies in the blood. My three grandchildren had negative screening tests, but one of their cousins screened positive. I was relieved about my grandchildren but still concerned about my son-in-law. It seemed curious that both type 1 and type 2 diabetes had suddenly appeared in the family.

Peter received appropriate medical treatment for a person newly diagnosed with type 2 diabetes. Metformin, an oral medication that lowers blood sugar, was prescribed. He was referred to a diabetes nurse educator who stressed proper nutrition. She introduced him to counting the grams of carbohydrates he ate, and recommended that he limit carbohydrates to sixty grams per meal. A one-ounce slice of regular bread contains about fifteen grams of carbohydrate.

"I don't like carbohydrate counting," Peter told me a few months after his diagnosis. "Before diabetes, eating was a straightforward process. It was never this much of an effort. Now it's a consuming and cumbersome process. I don't enjoy eating at all now."

At first he totally eliminated pasta and rice because he was afraid to eat them. After his diabetes educator reassured him that it was OK to take them in small portions, he became willing to eat a fistful of pasta now and then. "I don't touch french fries," he said, "and I only eat a small amount of popcorn a few times a week. The amount of popcorn I ate didn't have much to do with hunger, it was just a habit. Before diabetes, I had never been challenged to change my habits."

Peter lost twenty-five pounds the first two months, and has maintained his weight around 160 pounds subsequently. On the days when he doesn't play basketball or soccer, he jogs down the road (calling it his "medicinal three miles") or rides a stationary bicycle. He commented, "I don't like being stationary; I feel that if I pedal that hard, I should go somewhere."

His blood sugar levels after meals are usually normal now. He eats monster salads, often twice daily. The last time we went to a hockey game, I noticed no nachos between periods. "Giving up fast foods at sporting events was an easy one," he related. "But when I go out, I worry about hidden carbohydrates in the food. I think about it before, during, afterward." His blood sugar still goes above 200 mg/dl after pizza. "The guidelines say that a four-inch slice of pizza should contain only thirty grams of carbohydrate," Peter lamented. "I don't understand pizza. Counting carbs is just a hassle. I would rather just undereat. I could go to zero carbs at meals, but that's not healthy either." He generally eats the same food at the same time every day.

Peter had read somewhere that carbohydrates in liquid form were worse than solids. "I probably should drop beer altogether, but I still have one a few times a week, just in defiance, because I enjoy it." When asked if his use of the word "defiance" indicated any anger toward his physician or diabetes educator, he replied, "They're trying to help me; they give me clear guidelines, and I have the option to follow them. I get frustrated only by my relation to the diabetes, not by their role. Eating is a chore now—more of a battle than a pleasure. It used to be an activity without a counterpart. There's a perception that I'm struggling against a counterpart or an enemy."

For several months after his diagnosis, he seemed more solemn and didn't joke as much, but two years later, Peter said that he has gotten into a comfort zone about being forced to change his habits. He's more knowledgeable about nutritional issues and is more aware of his capabilities. His previous joviality has returned. However, I still hear subdued resentment and a resigned fatalism in his voice when he discusses diabetes. He recently had to begin insulin treatment, because his average blood sugar had increased to above target level. "I had been told that insulin treatment might be inevitable, but in the back of my mind I hoped I could put it off forever," he said. "My initial reaction was that I had done something wrong, but upon reflection I was doing exactly as I was instructed. Now my struggle is that even if I control my habits, I'm going to get worse. I thought I was doing a good job with my regimen, yet I still had to go on insulin. It's the nature of the disease—there are still elements I can't control. And I understand my risks of kidney disease, cardiovascular issues, complications."

I understood Peter's disappointment. His changes in eating and activity probably would have prevented the worsening of diabetes and the need for insulin therapy if he had typical type 2 diabetes. But he is representative of a subset of adults, initially diagnosed with type 2 diabetes, who show evidence of a slowly progressive form of autoimmune disease characterized by the presence of low levels of antibodies directed at the islet cells of the pancreas. This form of diabetes is called *latent autoimmune diabetes of adults* (LADA). Peter hadn't failed in his attempts to control diabetes: the progressive nature of his disease was more likely related to progressive destruction of his islet cells than to his lack of lifestyle changes.

Peter added, "I could have made the argument that diabetes was an opportunity—that in many ways my lifestyle habits are better and that I'm healthier than I have been in years—but emotionally it doesn't feel that way. Even if I get my diabetes under control, there's this invisible counterpart. It doesn't surprise me that there are lots of people who have a hard time managing diabetes."

Peter has been very public about discussing diabetes and insisted that his own name be used in this narrative. "It's important for people to talk about diabetes," he said, "I make an effort to build a network of support. It's not hard to get support from family and friends. You don't have to feel isolated or different. Everyone at work knows I have diabetes. This is the time of year the Easter candy comes, but they bring me almonds instead of chocolate bunnies. That comes from being open about it."

On a recent visit, I offered to take the family out to dinner and asked Peter to choose the restaurant. "That requires some thought and planning," he replied. "When it comes to eating, we have a complicated family, with two vegetarians, one diabetic, and one child whose entire menu consists of six items. I like a place with salads, but some like Chinese restaurants. Chinese is hard to manage because they usually don't have salads." The problem was solved when it was decided that the grandparents would take the grandchildren out for sushi, and Peter and my daughter would go on a date and have a quiet dinner alone.

Diabetes can have unanticipated effects on the family. Peter's eight-year-old son Saul said to me, "Grandpa, if I had all the money in the world, I would give it away to find a cure for diabetes."

CHAPTER 13

Who's in Control?

"I took control from the start—as soon as I came out of the hospital. I gave my own insulin shots; I weighed all my food. My parents didn't have a clue about diabetes, but my mother tried to take over control of my eating. This created a conflict for us." Allison, now a successful practicing physician in a large southern city, adds, "My parents and I are very close. They would love to talk to you about me."

Her mother, a slim, gracious woman now in her seventies, concurs: "We never gave her a shot; they taught her to do that in the hospital. When she came home, she was eating 2,400 calories a day and gaining weight. Seeing her able to consume so much food scared me. I am a woman; I have always valued beauty and appearance, and obesity is repulsive to me. It's within a person's ability to control."

Allison and each of her parents are consistent in their recollections, in their frank acknowledgment of the problems that diabetes has caused in their family, and in how they have reconciled their differing attitudes over twenty-five years.

During a youth choir bus trip at age fifteen, Allison had developed intense thirst and frequent urination, typical symptoms of uncontrolled diabetes. The girls on the trip had labeled her the "Pee Queen" because of her frequent trips to the bathroom.

Her mother recalls, "Learning that Allison had juvenile diabetes was the biggest shock of my life. I knew it could not be. Starting that 2,400 calorie diet in the hospital was the worst. I wondered what I might have done wrong. Was it because I had gained forty-five pounds during my pregnancy? After that day, I never baked another pie or cake."

Allison's father recalls, "When Allison returned home from the hospital, she was meticulous in her control of diabetes. Just once, when she hesitated to give herself a shot, I told her to put the insulin syringe between the door and the wall and just run into it. But Allison's high-calorie diet made my wife flip out."

Her mother has always felt people should be disciplined. "There's no need to be eating all the time. They should have some cereal and coffee for breakfast, a sandwich and a piece of fruit for lunch, meat and two vegetables for dinner, and that's it." Her husband says that if he opens the refrigerator door for an evening snack, she can hear it from the bedroom upstairs, and she shouts down, "Why do you need more food now? We had dinner."

"Insulin seemed to increase my appetite," maintains Allison. "I was always afraid of an insulin reaction at night, which led to habitual nighttime overeating. I ate at all hours of the night. The next morning my blood sugar would be high." Many physicians do not appreciate the frequency of low blood glucose levels during the night. Overeating at the time of low blood sugar is common and may lead to rebound higher blood sugar the following morning or contribute to weight gain.[1]

Allison thinks her mother considers being overweight a sin. "My mother's emphasis on controlling my weight led to problems with my image and self-esteem," she says. Her mother responds, "I think Allison has an eating disorder. Even now, when we travel together or when she stays overnight at my house, I see evidence of eating at night, ice cream bowls in the sink."

Allison was able to control her weight until the clinical years of medical training when she was often on call at night. Sleep and eating schedules became irregular. During her first three months as a medical resident, fattening snacks were provided for the doctors in the hospital cafeteria during the evening. Her mother was horrified. "She was plump. She looked horrible. I was shocked, angry, and disappointed. Her diabetes has caused me more stress, worry, and sadness than anything in my life. I couldn't say a word or she'd bite my head off. She forbade me to speak about her weight. She can't stand reprimands or criticism. Once, when I mentioned her weight, she grabbed my hair and shook it."

Allison's parents relate other aspects of dealing with the strong-willed teenager who evolved into an accomplished professional woman: "We always acquiesced to her needs. If we were on a trip, we ate when she was hungry and where she wanted to eat. She became selfish and used diabetes to manipulate others. Her mood swings were a demon and a curse. The family watchword became 'Don't upset Allison.'" Allison agrees with her parents and volunteers that her older brother says she uses diabetes "as an excuse to behave like a bitch."

Allison points out that growing up with diabetes influenced her choice of career. She has opened a holistic weight-management program to work in tandem with her medical practice. "I feel that I'm doing what I was destined to do. The biggest challenge for all persons with diabetes is to live your life like you would if you didn't have it," says Allison.

A few years ago, Allison started working with a personal trainer who challenged her. "I felt that if I was paying him sixty dollars, he should kick my butt," she says. "Although I had liked aerobics just to be-bop around, I had never been an athlete." She started running and training with a group of women and completed a marathon at age thirty-seven. Now she runs up to six miles several times per week and is slim and trim again. Her mother is very proud.

"Understanding the influence of illness on the family necessitates understanding the family itself, not just the illness. When the family becomes the focus, it will be seen that illness influences relationships as profoundly as it does individuals."[2]

CHAPTER 14

God, Do Not Let Me Cry

*Many memoirs of illness are written by children
about parents or by parents about children,
recounting not only an illness but a family.*
—Rita Charon[1]

Mothers worry—especially mothers of children with diabetes. They worry every day and every night, and they continue to worry even after the children have grown up. "I never went to bed without my stomach knotting up about him," acknowledges Robert's mother, thirty-one years after her son was diagnosed with type 1 diabetes. "Our life revolved around this child, and everything he did depended on us. I remember the day—Robert was twelve years old. We were on a trip, and he seemed to go to the bathroom forever; then he would drink this huge glass of water. When we stopped at McDonald's, he said he didn't want anything to eat, just the biggest glass of water they had."

Her grandfather had had diabetes, so she knew the symptoms. The next day she took a specimen of Robert's urine to the doctor's office "for my peace of mind . . . and I [have] never had a moment's peace of mind since that day." She continues, "I had to go home and tell my son he had diabetes. It was devastating, but I didn't want him to know how devastated I was. I was afraid I was going to cry. Before I talked to Robert, I had a talk with God and said, 'Listen, God, I'm depending on you. Do not let me cry.'"

When she tried to tell Robert that he had diabetes, he covered his ears and walked away. She followed him from room to room. She remembers telling him, "Robert, this is our lot in life, and we'll deal with it. Everybody has some problem. This is our problem. You can do everything you want to do; you'll just have to do this, too."

"From then on," she says, "he was never upset another time. He was a wonderful child, never defiant or belligerent, he just accepted it. Nobody else in our town had a child with diabetes, no one in the school had diabetes, so no one knew what we were dealing with. I was determined that Robert wasn't going to be different from other children. That was a huge thing with me."

It was 1975. Their family doctor sent them to a specialist in Gainesville, Florida, but all she remembers from that visit was the physician warning Robert that he should never scuba dive. They didn't go back. Robert's parents drove to Panama City each month to attend a support group. His mother states, "I was desperate for that kind of support." They learned about a summer camp for diabetic children, but Robert didn't want to go to a camp

A daily insulin shot was prescribed, as was the custom during that period. "You had to take that shot and take the food to match it; you had to eat that lunch and eat that snack," his mother recalls. "We had to test the urine: mix two drops of urine with five drops of water in a little test tube. When it turned orange, it was called 'four plus'; when that orange color appeared, my stomach just knotted up, and I worried myself to death."

Searching for more information, the parents took Robert to the Joslin Clinic in Boston for ten days. "We met another mother there; her son was named Jimmy. She would take apart a Big Mac sandwich, weigh each part on a balance scale, then reassemble the sandwich before letting Jimmy eat it. If I had done that sort of thing, I wonder if it would have changed anything."

They began seeing an endocrinologist in Jacksonville, Florida—a five-hour drive from home. After several visits, the doctor said that Robert needed two insulin shots a day. His mother told the doctor, "Oh, no, we don't need two shots a day. That will just make it harder."

"The doctor took me into another exam room, cut off the lights, and shut the door, leaving me in the dark for fifteen minutes. When he returned, he asked if I had cooled off."

"You really don't want two shots a day, do you?" the physician said. "OK, we can handle it with one for a while."

Two days after returning home, she called the doctor, saying, "We're ready for those two shots a day now."

The doctor replied, "Well, Robert and I have been ready for a long time, we just had to wait for you."

"That doctor handled me pretty well," she admits. "But back then, those two shots a day was a huge thing for me. I know that now they take four shots a day, right from the start."

Robert did everything his peer group did. He never thought that he was particularly inconvenienced by diabetes, but his mother continued to worry about him, always concerned that his blood sugar might be too low. When he played high school football, his mother would discreetly send his father to the locker room at halftime with a sandwich for Robert. When he played on the baseball team, she would bring Gatorade to the whole team. The night before he left for college, she admitted to Robert, "I've lied to you all these years; you're really not normal. Now I have to tell you the truth. When I brought Gatorade to your whole baseball team, I was really bringing it so that you wouldn't have low blood sugar."

"I knew that, Mama," he said.

She says, "He tries to keep me from worrying, and I try to make him think I'm not worrying, but he knows me."

His parents agree that Robert does not consider himself abnormal. In college, he once had to write a paper about something in his life that had affected the whole family. He called home and proposed with a questioning tone, "I can't think of anything to write about. I guess I could write about when I got diabetes."

"I guess you could," his mother replied to him. "Do you remember how you had to eat snacks when you went hunting up the river with your father? Do you remember how we always were careful about eating on time, how we couldn't go to the movies late in the afternoon because it would delay supper? What about when you took an insulin shot in a public restroom at Disneyland, how we were concerned that someone would think you were shooting up drugs?"

Robert's mother now recalls, "I didn't want to bare my soul and tell him how bad it had affected me. I told his dad that Robert doesn't think anything he did was unusual, it was just a way of life for him. He'll tell you to this day that he has no problems—he's that kind of person."

Robert is forty-four now, married, and a father. "Even now, when he gets in my car, I ask him if he brought a Coke or something sweet with him," his mother admits. "But now I'm getting into the part that I've always worried about, eye and kidney problems. This has been on my mind all this time. When the doctor told me that Robert had diabetes, I thought, 'I can deal with this, but down the road is going to be my big problem.' Eye problems have been devastating. The worst thing is worrying about the kidneys. He deals with it and tries to get his mama to deal with it. He says that he'll probably need a kidney transplant eventually, but it'll be fine."

"You deal with what life hands you," Robert reminds his mother.

"Using the insulin pump the last few years has changed Robert's life," according to his mother. "It has freed him from always having to eat right on time. Now he tests his blood sugar ten or twelve times a day. Still, I called him the other night and said, "Why don't you take a piece of candy before you go to bed?""

Robert responded to his mother playfully, "I'll eat two M&M's. Will that satisfy you?"

"I'll always worry about him," she sighs.

CHAPTER 15

Every Moment of Every Day

The family was gathered around the television watching *Marcus Welby, MD*. During the episode, which featured the case of a child with diabetes, twelve-year-old Mary Kathryn popped up and announced, "I think that's what I've got, diabetes, that's why I'm so thirsty."

She had been to church camp. When she returned, she looked like she had lost some weight. Her mother, concerned, called the mother of another girl who had been to camp, and was told that Mary Kathryn's friend had also lost a little weight; it was probably the camp food. Then the thirst began. The day after the television program, now thirty-two years ago, the doctor confirmed, "I think she does have diabetes. It's either diabetes or cancer."

At the hospital, Mary Kathryn's blood sugar was 750 mg/dl. A blood sugar level above 200 mg/dl, in the presence of symptoms such as Mary Kathryn's, confirms the diagnosis of diabetes. Her mother, now a retired second grade teacher, recalls the initial education of the family at the hospital:

> My husband took off from work to attend the training sessions, and my mother came up from Florida. They told us that we had the best family support group and were the most conscientious and dedicated parents that ever went through the training sessions. At one point they called my husband and me aside and wanted to tell us what terrible complications, kidney failure and blindness, could happen. I felt like it was the end of the world—so many dire predictions. They led us to believe that Mary Kathryn might not live to age thirty and probably would never be able to have children. I told them that they should tell Mary Kathryn exactly like it is. She's twelve years old and she can understand. They did, and she took it seriously. Right from

the start, she wanted to do what was right to take care of herself, but it took away the carefree parts of her life. She couldn't do the spontaneous things any more; it wasn't that easy a life any more.

She couldn't just suddenly decide to go on a picnic. If she wanted to spend the night with someone, we had to plan, we had to schedule everything; we had to be sure she had the insulin; we had to be sure she could test the urine; we had to be sure the people there could provide her with the proper food.

Her brother was in high school football at the time. I sort of pushed him aside and totally concentrated on Mary Kathryn for a while. We thought that never having sweets in the house didn't seem fair to my son; we decided to give him money to buy sweets when he was out.

"When there's a problem in my family," Mary Kathryn explains, "we take care of it as a family. We all learned how to give shots and how to treat low blood sugar. When diabetes was brand new, my mother was overprotective for a short time, but by the next year I tried out for the basketball team. Mom and I went to meet the coach and all the teachers. I didn't want to be treated differently. I played basketball and ran cross-country. My parents supported me by not making a big thing about it."

Her mother says further, "Mary Kathryn does such a good job of handling it herself that we forget about it. I compare our family with that of my best high school friend, whose daughter, the same age as Mary Kathryn, also developed diabetes as a child. Diabetes became my friend's whole life. She and her husband divorced; I think it was because she was totally focused on diabetes. Now, with her daughter age forty-three, diabetes is still all my friend talks about."

Nevertheless, Mary Kathryn admits that diabetes touches everything in her life:

You have to pay attention to it all the time. I have burned out at times, but you never get away from it. If you ignore it, you pay a price. Every day is about problem-solving and making constant decisions and choices. Each blood sugar level represents the end result of a situation where I had to make a choice.

Sometimes I take insulin before a meal; then I take a bite and find that it tastes horrible. Now I have to decide what to do.

If suddenly I had to leave my office for a fire drill, I would have to anticipate how far I needed to walk. Would the elevators be running? Would I be late for lunch? If I walked down six flights of steps, my blood sugar would drop from 90 mg/dl [normal] to 60 mg/dl [subnormal], and I'd need my glucose tablets.

If I go rollerblading with my son two miles from home, I must plan on ways to avoid low blood sugar. What if one of the rollerblade wheels broke and I had to walk home, and it took longer than usual?

While explaining the need to anticipate every scenario, Mary Kathryn cites the example of preparing a safe room for her family to use during the unexpected eventuality of a tornado. In addition to stocking the room with food, beverages, flashlights, and other survival equipment, she has to include insulin, supplies for her insulin pump, glucose tablets, and paraphernalia for blood glucose monitoring.

She frequently uses the word "constant" to discuss preparedness for unplanned events. During the flight to Cancun on her honeymoon, she noticed that she had failed to bring her glucose test strips. In addition to having a brand-new husband, being in a foreign country, and eating unfamiliar food, she felt panic in not knowing her blood sugar level. Ordinarily, she would have checked her blood sugar at least six or seven times each day. The couple spent the first three days of their honeymoon trying to find a pharmacy that could provide glucose test strips.

Mary Kathryn had experienced twenty years of diabetes treatment before using the insulin pump. She obtained her first pump twelve years ago, at the time of her first pregnancy. "I came from a different world of diabetes. I tested my urine before blood sugar monitoring was available, and I used the old insulins. The need to eat at specified times was so incredibly annoying. Having to eat the same amount of carbs at lunch every day was crazy—so unnatural. It went against the normal flow of daily life. When we got blood glucose meters, I thought it was the greatest gift. Then we got better types of insulins which were more predictable and decreased the constant fear of low blood sugar. Finally, the insulin pump has been my ticket to freedom. I can choose when to eat and the content of my meals. I can control high blood sugar quickly. Blood glucose monitoring and the pump have given me the opportunity to be normal. The truth is I survived before these luxuries—twenty years when we had nothing."

She says that her biggest advantage has been the support she has received both at home and at work. Mary Kathryn has firm ideas about what constitutes support. "My parents, brothers, husband, and kids never say, 'You shouldn't do that; you shouldn't eat that.' If I get that from anyone, it drives me insane. I know what I have to do; no one has to tell me. If my blood sugar is low, my husband or my children will get my meter and ask if I want to test my blood sugar, or they'll offer to get me some glucose tablets. That's support."

Once, at a staff meeting, carrot cake was served, and she decided to take a small piece. A colleague noticed her eating it and told Mary Kathryn she should not be eating cake. The intrusion infuriated her. On another occasion, when she was offered cake and refused it, someone said that even though she had diabetes, it would be OK for her to have a little.

When we asked what the word "control" meant to her, Mary Kathryn replied, "I have to deal with diabetes every day, but diabetes is not the controlling force in my life. Control not only means keeping my blood sugar in a certain range. It also means establishing who is in control. I am."

CHAPTER 16

It's Not About the Mom, It's About the Baby

Pregnancy is a condition that predisposes women to diabetes. When diabetes or elevated blood sugar is first recognized during pregnancy, it is called gestational diabetes (GDM). All women should be screened for GDM at twenty-four to twenty-eight weeks of pregnancy, which is around the beginning of the final three months.

There was no history of diabetes in Carolyn's family, so her screening positive for GDM was a big surprise. She wasn't terribly upset, however. "In your first pregnancy, you're so involved in the pregnancy and in having your first child, all the big dreams, you don't realize the significance of gestational diabetes," she said. After GDM was diagnosed, she took insulin and followed a diet closely. "I had always been a sweet-tooth person," she said. "I called it my sugar monster, and the more I fed it, the more it grew and wanted. It was a big adjustment not to eat sweets."

She required a cesarean section instead of a natural vaginal delivery. "The newborn baby was healthy," she said, "but later that night he developed low blood sugar. He didn't respond to the sugar water they gave him in the nursery." In the middle of the night, the baby was moved to the newborn intensive care unit, where he responded to IV glucose.

After Carolyn's delivery, her blood sugars returned to normal. "I went back to eating anything I liked," she recalled.

Four years later, GDM recurred. Carolyn related, "At the time of a routine monthly visit, my obstetrician said, 'With your history of GDM in the first pregnancy, we'll check you earlier than usual,' and of course I failed the screening test, and then I failed the three-hour glucose tolerance test again. I had already been through the excitement of having a child, so this time I took it more seriously. I knew what to expect. It's not about the mom, it's about the baby."

GDM usually resolves after delivery, only to return during subsequent pregnancies. Hormones produced by the placenta block the action of insulin in the mother's body. To compensate, a pregnant woman may need as much as three times as much insulin as a nonpregnant woman. Normal pregnant women can increase the production of insulin to meet this demand, and their blood sugar remains normal. A woman with subnormal capacity to secrete insulin may develop high blood sugar during pregnancy (gestational diabetes).

Pregnant women who don't have diabetes have blood sugar levels below 95 mg/dl in the fasting state before breakfast, below 140 mg/dl one hour after meals, and below 120 mg/dl two hours after meals.[1] Therefore, it is recommended that pregnant women with diabetes have similar home blood sugar levels. Regarding these requirements, Carolyn said, "I was upset at first. I asked, 'Why do you want my blood sugar below 100 mg/dl in the morning?" I was frustrated until I got my facts straight. I am trying to work full-time. I have to check my blood sugar at least six times a day, before I eat and an hour after I eat. It's a second job. I feel like I have a ball and chain."

High blood sugar, even in mild forms of GDM, is associated with abnormal outcomes involving the infant. A "fat baby"—one more than nine or ten pounds at birth (macrosomia)—is the most common newborn abnormality resulting from GDM. A large fetus increases the possibility that a cesarean section will be required.

Now Carolyn has two major concerns. The first involves her risk of having a big baby.

> But my biggest concern is that I might continue to have diabetes after this baby. It's kind of scary when you're doing insulin four times a day during pregnancy, and you think about having to take insulin or pills for diabetes long-term. At first my little four-year-old didn't want to be in the same room when I tested my blood sugar; he was scared of it. "Don't do it, Mom," he would say. Now he comes and watches me and pushes the button; he's part of it.
>
> When the baby was in the nursery after the first delivery, I thought, "I'll have a baby shower and eat cake, and if my blood sugar is elevated, that's OK." This time, I know I will need to

continue better eating habits and exercise after pregnancy. Now I'm more focused on my family. Am I going to be there for them? Do I want my four-year-old to grow up and know mom has to give herself shots? That is bothersome. I know the choices that I make for myself also will affect the family.

My family is in a transition. We sold our home, and we're building a house. We're temporarily living with my eighty-year-old grandmother. She doesn't understand why I'm taking shots, so she asks over and over. She went to the grocery store and filled up the whole pantry with sweets. We're living in one bedroom, and the baby crib will be there. We have been eating out a lot, so we have our family time and quiet time from my grandmother. When I heard I had GDM again, I thought, "Oh, now I've got to cook." I grew up with gravies, biscuits, sausage, bacon. I learned to cook that way. I had finally learned to make really good gravy, and now it's probably not the best thing to do.

Long-term follow-up studies show that most women who have gestational diabetes do eventually develop diabetes. Thus, gestational diabetes can be viewed as an early stage of diabetes in evolution.[2]

CHAPTER 17

I Need to Hear His Voice

Anne describes attending a dinner party where she witnessed Pat, another guest, sitting in a corner of the room frantically speaking into her cell phone. "She dialed and redialed, leaving messages: 'Where are you? Call me. Where are you? Call me back.' Only after her husband, Jim, arrived about thirty minutes later, after a late meeting at work, did Pat relax and put her phone away."

Pat was appropriately concerned. Her husband had type 1 diabetes and a history of problems with severe hypoglycemia. Hypoglycemia is normally accompanied by obvious warning signs: weakness, trembling, sweating, and lightheadedness. These symptoms are a blessing in disguise. In response to the warning, a food or liquid with simple sugar is consumed, blood sugar rises back to normal, and the symptoms resolve. However, some people who have lived with diabetes for many years lose these early warning signs. Jim had had diabetes since age nine. He had unawareness to hypoglycemia. In this situation, the blood sugar can drop dangerously low. The brain is unable to function normally without glucose.

Severe hypoglycemia is defined as low blood glucose resulting in stupor, seizure, or unconsciousness that makes self-treatment impossible. It is the primary barrier to intensive insulin treatment of diabetes.[1] Repeated episodes of coma due to unawareness to hypoglycemia tyrannize the life of the patient and his loved ones. Jim had often been found unconscious. "When we first married, I knew he had hypoglycemia unawareness," Pat explained later, "but he had not had any scary episodes yet. When I call him and he doesn't answer the phone, that scares me. That's the underlying current of how diabetes affects our marriage."

According to Pat, the scariest episode of severe hypoglycemia occurred when Jim was driving a truck with a trailer on the interstate.

At noon, he had given himself his insulin but had failed to eat lunch. In all likelihood, he had realized that something was wrong, because he pulled over to the side of the road, but he couldn't hang on to consciousness. The wheels of his truck were turned away from the interstate. His foot slipped off the brake, allowing the truck and the trailer to slide down the embankment onto a long grassy shoulder in front of some trees at the bottom of the incline. Somebody noticed the reflective tape on the back of his trailer and called the police.

Jim remembers very little about the episode except waking when the EMTs arrived. He remembers reaching for his glucose tablets in the glove compartment, but the EMTs thought he was reaching for a gun or drugs. He doesn't wear a necklace or bracelet to indicate he has diabetes, because he's afraid it will catch in equipment in his work.

Pat says:

> The police called me about 7 p.m., reporting that Jim was at the emergency room at Murfreesboro. His blood sugar had dropped to 30 mg/dl. He had tried to call during the episode, but in the confusion of hypoglycemia he had evidently called my office phone instead of the phone at home. The next day at work I found a voicemail message that had recorded Jim's hollering, the EMTs talking and checking his blood sugar, and the struggle to remove him from the truck.
>
> Jim works as a landscape contractor, so he's physically active all day, but he can out-work all the strategies that he knows to keep his blood sugar from getting too low. His biggest risk time is between 5 and 7 p.m. He'll get back from whatever job he's been doing, they were trying to beat the dark or beat the rain tomorrow, whatever, and it's been the longest since he's had anything to eat.
>
> Once I called him and said, "Hey, when are you coming home?" I got no response. After several tries, I yelled, "Where are you?" Then he answered, "I'm here." "Where?" "I'm here," and I knew instantly his blood sugar was low, that he wasn't in his right mind, and I had no idea where he was.
>
> His dad, our friends Dave and Sue, and everybody got out on the road looking for him. By the time I got to town, his dad and Sue had discovered him parked at his storage lot behind an eight-foot fence with barbed wire on top. They could see him

sitting in his truck slumped over the steering wheel. Showing what fear can do for added strength, his dad actually scaled the fence, while Sue yelled from the other side, "Find the glucose tablets, find the glucose tablets." By the time I got there, Jim was better, but he couldn't drive home.

Pat says the hardest part of being Jim's spouse is not the cooking or the diet. "If he didn't have hypoglycemia unawareness, diabetes wouldn't be much of an issue. He's never angry or impatient or upset, so if he is, I know his blood sugar is low. I'll just hand him glucose tablets and not even address the fact that he might need it. That doesn't work if he's coming out of sleep at night; he's combative then. He'll throw away the glucose tablets or he'll put them in his mouth but not chew them—like a six-year-old."

Pat advises other spouses whose husbands have diabetes to talk about it candidly:

You need to know how the person with diabetes wants to handle it. Does he want help? What kind of help? Find out what pushes each other's buttons about diabetes. My husband told me not to ask if his blood sugar is low. "Just hand me something to eat" is his preference. If I didn't know how he felt about it, I would make the situation worse.

When he was preparing for his busy season, I told him he needed to be more considerate of my feelings. "If you have an appointment at 7 p.m., tell me. If you don't call me, and I can't reach you, you know what happens in my mind. Not knowing where you are, or if you're safe, makes me worry. It's not just that I'm afraid; I'm looking out for you, too."

If Jim had a desk job and wasn't so physical during the day, and if he didn't hunt deep in the woods, and if he didn't go on those wilderness canoe trips, living with diabetes would be nothing. I don't know how I survived the first years of marriage before cell phones. I insisted we buy cell phones before he thought he needed one, just for peace of mind. I wanted to be able to communicate with him, just touch base and hear his voice to know that he is OK.

Recently the technological advance of continuous glucose monitoring has been introduced into clinical care of diabetes. A tiny sensor is inserted under the skin and held in place by an adhesive. The sensor monitors the glucose level in the surrounding tissue and wirelessly transmits the data to a receiver that can be worn or hand-held. With the push of a button, the patient can view his current blood sugar level, as well as recent trends in the levels. Also, the receiver can sound an alarm for high or low glucose levels, prompting corrective action.

The following narrative illustrates some of the advantages and limitations of this new technology.

Bridget is a fifty-nine-year-old math and science teacher who has had type 1 diabetes for thirty-eight years. "Diabetes controls your life," she asserts.

I have lots of hypoglycemia. I get confused a few times every day, and I pass out once or twice a month. I've had five car wrecks caused by hypoglycemia. After one accident I was kept in the drunk tank at jail for five hours. The Breathalyzer tests showed no alcohol, and I don't drink. Once, my driver's license was revoked for six months.

When my children were little, I had so much hypoglycemia that I had a nanny—not for them, for me—because my husband wouldn't let them be with me alone.

Except for hypoglycemia, I have no complications from diabetes and haven't been in a hospital for thirty years. I lock horns with Kathleen, my diabetes nurse practitioner, because I think I'm as much an authority on diabetes as she is. I try too hard to keep my blood sugar normal, that's why I overshoot. She gets on me when she sees all those low blood sugars. She wants me to lower the rate of insulin on my insulin pump. I'm not a doctor, but I know me. I'm terrified of high blood sugar, because it will damage my eyes and kidneys. I'm not terrified by low blood sugar, even if I pass out. I always come around, and hypoglycemia doesn't cause permanent damage to my body like high blood sugar does.

Bridget acquired a continuous glucose monitor recently. At the time of this interview, she had used the system for two months. During the two hours we spent together, she checked the display of her blood sugar level at least a dozen times. "It's totally changed my life," she relates. "I feel more independent. I haven't felt that way since the onset of diabetes. Even my mother believes in it. I can work in the yard longer, I can shop longer, I can teach without stopping, I can stay at school longer. I have less anxiety, I feel more confident. The hypoglycemic reactions at night have gone away. My A1c test improved, indicating improvement in my average blood sugar."

The new monitor hasn't changed everything, however. "It beeps four or five times each day. Sometimes when I'm teaching I hear the beep and just turn it off. Last week, the kids in my class said, 'You're beeping.' I heard them, but I did nothing. I lost consciousness in the classroom; it was my own fault. My husband and son had to come to school. When they tested my blood sugar, it was very low. I had set the alarm to go off at 85 mg/dl, and it beeped. I had four alarms and didn't respond to them. Even before I had the sensor, I would get confused and not respond when others in my presence would indicate to me that my blood sugar was low. If I don't respond to the alarms, how is this wonderful new gadget going to help me?"

Preliminary clinical research has indicated that continuous glucose monitoring systems are usually safe and accurate and correlate fairly well with results of fingerstick blood sugar monitoring. The alarms for low and high blood sugar give patients the opportunity to treat some problems of which they otherwise would have been unaware. The majority have overall improvements in blood glucose control and less time spent in both the low blood sugar and high blood sugar ranges.[2]

CHAPTER 18

Like Having a Partner

Sometimes family members monitor for hypoglycemia, as Pat does for Jim; in Bridget's circumstance, a continuous glucose monitor has helped; but Lisa has found another alternative—a new family member.

We met at a coffee house near the Vanderbilt campus. Zorrita entered first, followed closely by Lisa, who was holding the other end of the leash. Zorrita wore her blue service dog vest proudly; its pockets were packed full, like those of a Cub Scout going on a hike. Her short legs made her appear surprisingly small for a service dog with major responsibilities. I learned that she was part Labrador and part dachshund.

Lisa was smiling and exuberant. I remembered her as a patient whose life had been miserable because of frequent episodes of sudden hypoglycemic coma. She is fifty-four now, "after forty-four years of this damn disease," she reminded me.

"About ten years ago, I started losing my warnings for hypoglycemia," Lisa recounted. "My blood sugar could go from 350 mg/dl to 40 mg/dl in 1½ hours. I would suddenly pass out with no warning. EMTs were coming to my house to revive me with intravenous glucose several times a month. We got the continuous glucose monitor, but since it monitors interstitial fluid instead of blood, it wasn't fast enough. It had a twenty minute lag, which was enough time for me to get foggy. By the time the monitor alarm sounded, I was already out of it. When the blood sugar was dropping fast, ten to fifteen minutes could make a huge difference in whether I passed out or not."

A former professor of Spanish who speaks five languages, Lisa described how she felt after recovering from an episode of coma due to low blood sugar. "I would feel like my brain wasn't functioning well, and I worried that I was killing off brain cells. I used to be able to think fast and could balance all kinds of ideas and tasks at the same time. I got to the point where I didn't know if I would live much longer."

In the past year, Zorrita changed all that.

"Zorrita can smell differences in my blood sugar levels. Let's demonstrate how Zorrita would behave if it were low now." Lisa took a piece of cotton that had been soaked in her saliva at a time when her blood sugar was low, then frozen for use in training. She put the cotton in her mouth. Within seconds, Zorrita snapped to attention, took up a position immediately in front of Lisa, stared intensely at her, and began to lick her face. "You're licking me a lot, do you think my blood sugar is low?" asked Lisa. Zorrita persisted. "Find the meter. Find the meter," Lisa instructed. Zorrita ran to her purse and returned with her blood glucose meter. "Good girl."

"She can tell my blood sugar is abnormal just from sniffing my hands," Lisa explained. "She likes to sniff my mouth, but she can make do with my hands. When she actually smells the blood and is certain that the blood sugar is low, she knows, 'This is not OK.'"

Lisa pricked her finger tip. "It's low—find the sugar, find the sugar," Lisa instructed. Zorrita ran to her purse and returned with the bottle of glucose tablets. "When I have a low blood sugar, she'll stare at me and not rest until we do the whole routine and I eat the glucose tablet. Sometimes she will get the glucose tablets if I'm a little foggy and don't even tell her. Now I'll eat a glucose tablet, then Zorrita will get her treat for finding a low blood sugar. It's a graham cracker, her favorite food. It's her 'find a low' treat."

After eating the graham cracker, Zorrita relaxed and took a quick nap at our feet. After several minutes, I asked Lisa if Zorrita could check my blood sugar. I was instructed to hold my hand in front of her nose and say, "Check me." Zorrita sniffed my hand and walked away, uninterested. "You're boring to her since your blood sugar is normal," Lisa explained.

Zorrita can also detect high blood sugar. "If my blood sugar is high, she'll lick and pester me," Lisa said. "She gives me the same signal for both low and high blood sugar, but for training I give her a different treat for each. I haven't bothered to train her to give me different signals for high and low blood sugar, because I always have a meter around. I wear a continuous glucose monitor, so I don't depend much on Zorrita for high blood sugar. The monitor has been more helpful for me for highs than for lows. Since low blood sugar is followed by horrendous bounces to high blood sugar, my average blood sugar was usually high, and the lowest A1c test I could achieve was 8.1 percent. Within three months of acquiring Zorrita and preventing severe hypo-

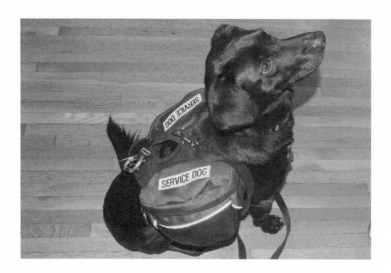

Zorrita on duty

glycemia, my A1c test had fallen to 7.6 percent, and my overall blood sugar has been less volatile and better controlled."

Lisa acquired her service dog from Pawsibilities Unleashed Pet Therapy in Frankfort, Kentucky. The organization had trained the dog to react to blood glucose scents; then Lisa went to Kentucky for a week, where she was taught how to continue Zorrita's training. After she returned home, she trained Zorrita to retrieve her meter from her purse, and she has continued to enhance her dog's skills.

Liz Norris, the founder of Pawsibilities Unleashed, is an animal behaviorist with more than thirty years of dog training experience, including K-9 obedience in the U.S. Air Force. "When you've trained a dog to detect a dangerous gas leak twenty feet underground or to rescue a fallen comrade in crossfire, training service dogs is natural," she says.

One of Liz's clients with diabetes sleeps in a t-shirt. She calls him her Living Scent Source. When his blood sugar is high or low, he peels off the t-shirt and puts it in a Ziploc, labels it with his blood sugar level, and freezes it. At animal shelters, she offers little pieces of the t-shirts to the dogs, looking for the ones who respond to the abnormal blood sugar scent by becoming very alert: the scent seems to bother them. The exact sensory cue to the dogs' awareness is not known, but most evidence points to their ability to detect scents in the person's body and clothing. Even untrained dogs have detected hypoglycemia in their owners before any symptoms were noticed, and canine sensing of glucose in patients with diabetes has become more sophisticated thanks to behavioral training.[1]

Liz looks for dogs with kind temperaments and a heightened sense of smell. During the training process, she refines their natural ability by offering rewards for appropriate behavior. For the dogs, it's a game, because they receive treats and lots of positive reinforcement after a correct alert.[2]

I asked Lisa how her life has changed since she acquired Zorrita. She replied, "Having Zorrita is like having a partner in managing diabetes. She monitors my disease 24/7; she's always interested, always concerned, always helping me with it." She continued, tearfully, "It's a gift: it's like someone holding your hand and being so concerned. It lifts some of the burden in a way that's hard to quantify or even describe."

Lisa has not lost consciousness since Zorrita has joined her family:

> Zorrita can recognize when a rapid drop in blood sugar is occurring, even when my blood sugar is still in the normal range, and alerts me to treat the condition before it turns into a crisis. She is always right. She won't take no for an answer. She'll lie down but keep staring at me; in a few minutes, she'll start pestering me again. She's earlier and more accurate in telling me when my blood sugar is dropping than my continuous glucose monitor. She is real-time. And the most wonderful thing is that I'm starting to recognize symptoms of hypoglycemia again.
>
> I'm still working with Zorrita on what to do if I'm unconscious. I'm going to train her to go and get someone. These dogs can be trained to dial 911, using a special pad that attaches to the phone. She doesn't alert me when my husband Doug is home. She feels he's in charge then, and she's not on duty. She seems to think Doug is the alpha dog.

Service animals are legally defined in the Americans with Disabilities Act of 1990, and federal laws protect the rights of individuals with disabilities to be accompanied by their service animals in public places.

PART III

The Social Context of Control

In many instances, the critical element of diabetes control is not the patient's autonomy, the family, or the clinician–patient relationship, but the social context. Social relationships can outweigh all other influences.

The dominant factor influencing diabetes may come from the circumstances of one's daily life. A situation at school, in the workplace, at a recreational site, or in the health care system may become the prevailing effect on a patient's control of diabetes.

The environment can be a powerful determinant as well. Exposure to chemicals in the environment may influence or even cause diabetes, and a disaster such as a hurricane can have an enormous effect on diabetes control.

Moreover, the availability of medical and social resources impacts diabetes control. The country in which one lives—even the neighborhood—can influence the course of diabetes. The move from a rural to an urban lifestyle, and the process of migration to a country with better economic opportunities, are often serious determinants of diabetes control.

CHAPTER 19

It's a Bet

At age fifty-four, Morrie is a successful attorney. His diabetes was diagnosed about eleven years ago, but its control has been limited by his excessive weight.

Morrie had gone to a nutritionist, but he said he knew how to count calories; the visits weren't helpful. He had tried Weight Watchers twice. "I had good success the first three weeks," he said. "I lost about fifteen pounds. I went to the meetings, I was bragging. All the women there hated my guts; they had been struggling for months. After that initial loss, I couldn't lose more weight. I stopped the program."

His mother had once enticed him to lose weight by offering to buy him three new suits. "I won the bet," he recounted. "I got the suits, but it was just to lose a few pounds."

Then several years ago, his friend Mel suggested that they enter a bet to see who could lose the most weight in four months. Their friendship wasn't based on gambling. Their children and wives were friends, and they had gone on vacations together. Morrie explained:

Although neither of us had diabetes at that time, we were both destined to become diabetic. Mel and I were about the same height, 5' 10", close in weight, about the 250–260 range. Mel was a successful gambler. For several years he had been playing in card games, not only in Nashville but in Tunica, Mississippi, and in Las Vegas. He consistently won. He's a good poker player. I am not a true gambler. I never liked going to Las Vegas. I've never left an organized gambling facility a winner, but I am more comfortable gambling on myself than on a horse race or a baseball game.

We decided that the loser of the bet would take both families to Destin, Florida, for a one-week vacation. The loser would pay for the lodging, the food, and the transportation. It was Mel's challenge. I lost fifty pounds in the four months. Mel lost about thirty-five pounds. Mel took the families to Destin, and we had a very nice time.

I asked Morrie how he did it. He replied:

The motivation was just the bet—pure competition. Back then, it was pretty easy. I had confidence and was in command from the start. I carefully watched what I ate; I calorie-counted, and I exercised excessively. I would dictate to my secretary on the treadmill, and I even had conversations with clients while I was walking on the treadmill. They would ask me why I was breathing so heavily, and I would say, "I'm exercising. I'm happy to take your call, but I'm going to keep exercising."

I'm a type A personality. I'm highly organized and highly competitive. Law is a competitive field, and advocacy is confrontational. I don't like to lose; I take professional losses personally. At the end of a lawsuit, I try to shake the other person's hand if he has done a good job, but I can tell you that if I lose, I'm not happy—for me or for my client.

The day after the bet, both bettors fell back into their old habits. Their caloric intake increased dramatically, and the exercise diminished similarly. In four or five months, both men had regained the weight and were back in the 250-pound range. By then, Mel had developed type 2 diabetes.

They initiated their second bet. Morrie lost fifty pounds and won again; Mel lost about thirty-five pounds. To celebrate the end of the bet, they went out to an Italian restaurant. Each had a veal parmigiana, and they split a third one. Then Mel took the couples to Lake Tahoe for a weeklong skiing vacation.

Now it's irritating Mel. He doesn't like to lose gambling—especially to me—it's driving him crazy. I keep reminding him of the two free vacations. Soon we start joking about how we're going to gain the weight back, so we can have the next bet. We fall back into our old habits and regain the weight.

By now Mel's diabetes is about to become insulin-dependent, and I have become diabetic too—about age forty-three. Mel is seven years older, and I trail him in a health pattern. I win the third bet, and Mel has to take me and my wife to Nassau, in the Caribbean. Now, Mel's wife is getting mad at him; it's been three vacations. They try to get us to do a combined husband-wife weight loss bet. Both wives are a little overweight, but not to the extent of their husbands. My wife is willing to go along, but I won't do it; I don't want to ruin my record. I don't want to take the risk of relying on my wife as a partner in a weight-loss bet. I win the fourth bet, again to Nassau. These are not inexpensive vacations—they each probably cost Mel about $6,000. For Mel, these are numbers he has lost at a poker table, but it's bothering him so much that I have beaten him four times. I would never gamble this amount of money.

The last weight-loss bet was about eight years ago. Mel had to pay for the airfare, lodging, food, and ski lifts for the two couples' ski trip to Snowmass, Colorado. Morrie won five out of five bets, each time losing about fifty pounds. "Mel thought he was close at the end of the last bet. The night before the final weigh-in, he slept in his car in a plastic wrestling suit, in an effort to lose body weight. That was the closest he came, but it didn't work. Now he weighs about 265, I'm about 230."

During the last bet, Morrie's A1c dropped from over 10 percent to 5.8 percent, indicating a decrease in average blood sugar from above 240 mg/dl to under 125 mg/dl. He was able to stop his anti-diabetic pills. He was eating as little as 1,000 calories on some days and was walking nine miles a day on his treadmill at three miles an hour, conducting business while walking. After he regained the weight, he had to start insulin, and is now taking 100 units daily.

Recently, Morrie initiated a weight-loss bet with his twenty-two-year-old daughter, whom he describes as having the same competitive streak as he. He said he competed with his daughter because he wanted her to lose weight. It wasn't the intense contest it had been with Mel. "I hired a personal trainer for both of us," he said. "We would go to the gym together twice a week and we made tremendous strides. For the first time, I enjoyed exercise. With Mel, I exercised just to win the bet, but now I exercise because I want to be healthy. I rarely miss a daily trip to the gym. I recently went on a two-week ski trip, during which I cross-country skied three of the days and I lifted weights. I skied better than I had in fifteen years. I was able to ski from the top of the mountain to the bottom without stopping."

In persons with genetic predisposition to type 2 diabetes, increased fat within the abdomen usually precedes the onset of diabetes. Increased abdominal fat leads to an apple-shaped appearance, in contrast to the pear-shaped appearance associated with increased fat in the hip area. In this country, abdominal obesity is defined as abdominal circumference greater than forty inches in men and greater than thirty-five inches in women.

Incorporating physical activity into daily living is the most useful strategy to maintain weight loss. The most common activity is brisk walking for about an hour per day. A goal of 10,000 steps per day is advocated for weight maintenance. Considering that the average American adult walks 3,000–5,000 steps per day, this may seem like a lot of walking to some people. After a baseline is established, it can be increased by about 20 percent each month to reach the goal of 10,000 steps daily. A step pedometer is helpful.

CHAPTER 20

Blown Away

Roberta left New Orleans the day before Hurricane Katrina struck. One of her sons drove her to her brother's home in Nashville, eight hours away and out of harm's reach. "I saw it only on TV," she acknowledged in an interview several months afterward.

My kids got caught up in it. It took almost three weeks before they were all located, but it seemed like months. I thank God they got me out of there, because I don't think I could have survived it. We had a problem getting out of town; the traffic was real bad. Thinking I could go home in a couple of days, I didn't bring anything with me except a couple of outfits. I didn't even bring my blood glucose meter, medication, or insulin. I was very nervous and shaky and upset. My diabetes pretty much went haywire.

I lived in the city, right off Canal and Broad in a four-bedroom, two-story home. I lived downstairs, and my son was staying with me in the rear. My daughter and her kids lived upstairs. They were rescued from my house, at first in a little boat; then a helicopter raised them up in the air and put them on a bridge on the interstate. They stayed on that interstate bridge for four days and three nights and eventually wound up in Texas. My daughter called when she got to Houston. They're doing fine now, but the four-year-old would get to howling and crying for a good while. Whenever the wind started blowing hard, he would get afraid, like we got another hurricane coming.

Before the hurricane, I was doing OK. I was being treated with insulin and Glucophage and Glucotrol pills for diabetes at Charity Hospital. I was taking insulin every day. After the hurricane, I missed just the first day. I went to Kmart in Nashville and the pharmacist there was nice enough to give me my medication until I could get to a doctor. My brother took me down to Vanderbilt Hospital about three days later. I saw a doctor and got prescriptions. There was no way to get in touch with the doctors back home.

Roberta relates, "My blood sugar was running high, but I didn't have a meter until I was here a month. It was probably higher, because, like the blood pressure, it has a tendency to be higher when you're upset. I couldn't sleep; I pretty much lost my appetite. I drank cokes and a lot of coffee, and I cried a lot."

When asked what was the most serious effect of the hurricane for her, Roberta says:

Losing everything I had accomplished in my adult life. I lost all my furniture, my jewelry, all my important papers, a lot of things that have sentimental value. It took a toll on me a good while; then I realized I was blessed to have my life. At fifty-seven years old, and disabled, I have a problem starting over. The kids, they are young, they can start over. My son has a home in La Vergne, Tennessee, now; he's doing good. My daughter is working, got the kids in nursery—but me, I'm stuck like Chuck.

We couldn't go back into the city for an extended time. When we returned, the house was all flooded and messed up, everything molded and mildewed. It stank. It had sat in that water for days; they say everything is contaminated. The water was up to the box spring in my bedroom downstairs, and the water was on the third step that leaves upstairs. There was a lot of wind damage up there, too.

They haven't renovated it yet. I had some very nice furniture. I was set for the rest of my life. I didn't bother with it, I just walked away and said, "Thank God we got our lives."

As a health care professional, Anne worked as a volunteer at a shelter in Nashville for Hurricane Katrina refugees, where one of the biggest problems was the patients' lack of knowledge regarding the names of their medications or the type of insulin they used. "The little white pill for high blood pressure" was not an unusual response. In addition, some individuals tried to abuse the system to obtain pain pills or tranquilizers that they could subsequently sell.

The story of Virginia, a chapter manager for the Red Cross in a small town in Middle Tennessee, illustrates another example of Hurricane Katrina's effect on diabetes patients. Virginia's job was part-time, and she was the only paid employee. She had speaking engagements every week at various civic organizations. She raised money locally and managed the office. There was always a turnover in volunteers, but she usually could count on about forty due to her active recruiting efforts.

Though she had always been slightly overweight, she managed her type 2 diabetes meticulously. She cooked a healthy dinner for her husband and herself every night, and they had time to enjoy Western dancing a few times each week. After dancing for three hours, sometimes her blood sugar would drop, and she'd have to sit down and get a snack, but life wasn't difficult for her until Hurricane Katrina hit New Orleans.

Within a few weeks, sixty-six displaced families had shown up in Virginia's small town. Regardless of their previous positions before the hurricane, these families now had no income and no place to stay. "They would call me at home as soon as they got to town," she said.

Virginia's life suddenly became stressful, because she felt responsible for the care of each family. "I wasn't trained for this," she explained. Though the job was supposed to be part-time, now she was working more than full-time, usually into the evening hours. "I quit eating right and taking care of myself. I was totally eating fast food, hamburgers, biscuits, stuff I hadn't eaten for years. Now even my husband was eating at fast food restaurants on the way home from work. He gained weight and developed a fatty liver."

She managed to settle almost all the sixty-six families in rental property donated by her fellow townspeople. "We had no shelters, and we spent only $3,500 on motels for a few families," she said. "I went on radio and TV and raised $48,000 locally, and the national Red Cross advanced our chapter $50,000. This was a lot of money for a usual annual budget of $25,000."

Almost six months after the hurricane, most of the sixty-six families have returned to New Orleans, and only a handful remain locally. "We have only twelve children from displaced families in school now," she announced proudly.

She had gained eighteen pounds, and her average blood glucose had increased considerably. "Now I'm going to start exercising again and eating dinner at home with my husband to get this diabetes back under control," she stated.

Stress is a potential contributor to uncontrolled diabetes. Stress stimulates hormones that mobilize glucose as energy for the "fight or flight" response. In persons with diabetes, the stress-induced increases in glucose cannot be used properly due to insufficient insulin; elevated blood sugar levels result.

Stress or depression may also be associated with abnormal eating behaviors. Patients with excessive eating in the evening hours may choose disproportionately large quantities of fat- and carbohydrate-rich foods, challenging self-care regimens that aim to regulate glucose levels.[1]

A study at three health care systems in New Orleans showed that Hurricane Katrina had significant adverse effects on diabetes management and on socioeconomic-related disparities in health.[2]

CHAPTER 21

Warrior Mode

Jeff has had type 1 diabetes for thirty-one years. "In my case, good control has resulted in virtually no complications," he said. "I check my blood sugar at least six times a day, sometimes more. I get at least an hour of exercise daily, more on weekends. But I do have issues with hypoglycemia, and my insulin pump is important to me. If I need anything other than insulin or syringes, I may have to fight to get it."

By fight, Jeff means battling his health insurance company. He's had lots of experience in this battle, from which he has drawn the following conclusions: "People in insurance companies are paid bonuses for cost containment. Their mission is to make a profit; I understand that. If what they say is not in writing in your plan, question it and make them verify, in writing, that whatever they're telling you is true. They may be just making it up, or somebody way down in the chain may tell you something just to make you walk away."

Jeff related some dramatic examples:

My first experience happened shortly after I started to work at a large employer. The health benefits plan came to me in the mail. It indicated that insulin pumps and the supplies for the pump were a covered benefit. I had an insulin pump at the time, but I was concerned about the monthly cost of the supplies (about $200). When I went to the benefits fair, I asked the representative of the health insurance company about insulin pumps, and she said, 'No, we don't cover insulin pumps.' I showed her the flyer which had been mailed to me, indicating that insulin pumps were covered, but she insisted that the company was not responsible for covering insulin pumps. I casually mentioned to her that since this document had come to me in the U.S. mail, if it wasn't honored, maybe we should investigate that as mail fraud. Within twenty-four hours, a meeting took place between the health insurance company and the director of benefits of my employer. That's how I got to know who the director of benefits was. Since then, I have e-mailed her about these matters, and I've always gotten a response within a day. During one fight, I called her office three times a day. Though I've never met her personally, she probably cringes when she sees my name.

A few years later, my pump gave me a warning that the warranty was about to expire. If my pump [was] to malfunction, and it was still under warranty, the pump company would send me a new one within twenty-four hours. If it malfunctioned after the warranty expired, I'd be out of luck. I knew I had to get a new pump. I called my health insurance company and was told that, if my pump was still functioning, I could only get a new one every five years.

Jeff asked me, as his physician, to write a letter to the medical director of the insurance company in his behalf, documenting that a new pump was medically necessary. I complied. When his request for a new pump continued to be denied, Jeff had to enter what he calls "Warrior Mode." He documented every conversation with any representative of the insurance company, typing while the conversation was taking place. Then he would read it back to the employee, adding, "You have said you do not replace pumps except every five years; have I heard you correctly? Please send me the written policy of the insurance company regarding this issue. Also, I need your first name and your employee ID number, for I'm going to quote you when I speak with the director of benefits at my company."

The medical director of the health insurance company denied his request for a new pump. He said a pump wasn't medically necessary, even though the insurance company had been providing pump supplies for Jeff for three years. Jeff asked for the medical director's name and direct telephone number and was told that information was not available. "Is that company policy?" Jeff asked, and was told that it was. He asked them to fax him a copy of that part of the company's policy but was told his request was impossible to fulfill.

"I had read the contract between my employer and the insurance company," said Jeff. "The department of benefits of my employer wouldn't give me a copy, but they let me read it in the Human Resources office. It goes into detail. If you're willing to sit in a very cramped space and go through hundreds of pages, you can find it, and

I did. Then I e-mailed the director of benefits. My point in dealing with the department of benefits was that if my insulin pump went down, it would take weeks for me to get a new one, and during that time my employer would be paying the emergency room bills." Jeff summarized all his hypoglycemic events and emergency room visits. He indicated that the new pump would have a glucose "wizard," making it easier to avoid low blood sugar. "I told her, 'You look at the cost of a pump and compare it with the cost of three emergency room visits.' The director of benefits replied to me that there was no requirement that I wait five years for a new pump."

On his next call to the insurance company, Jeff requested a case manager. He elaborated, "You have to fight to get a case manager; ordinarily you don't get one unless you're a complex case. Then my nurse, Anne, talked to my case manager. With the additional documentation that Anne gave them, they overturned the previous decision of the medical director in thirty-two minutes. The case manager told me to ignore the letter from the medical director. I never got a chance to talk with him, but I would have requested a doctor-to-doctor conversation. And I was considering filing a grievance with my director of benefits. It was extraordinarily time-consuming, involving 30–40 hours of my time. The calling and calling just wore them down, but it was the insurance company case manager who turned it around."

Jeff's health insurance company paid approximately $4,500 for his new pump; he was responsible for the 20 percent co-payment. His monthly out-of-pocket co-payment for pump supplies is about $75. His policy covers his glucose test strips as a prescription drug benefit, costing him only a $30 monthly copayment.

A few months after he got his new insulin pump, Jeff received a notice from his insurance company stating that insulin pump supplies were not a covered benefit. He called his case manager, and she promptly resolved that problem.

"I am one of several thousand people who call that insurance company daily. The people there are just doing their job as they have been instructed. When you are trying to get something, the more constructive noise you can make convinces them you are someone who knows his stuff, who can't just be pushed around like everyone else. That, with documentation, makes the difference," he said.

When Jeff goes into Warrior Mode, he is fighting more than a bureaucrat at his health insurance office. He is fighting a system—a system of financing health care. One of the goals of this system is to restrict health care costs. For most workers in the United States, most of these costs are paid by an employer and constitute a business expense. If health care costs are high, the profits are reduced, or the price of the product of the workers' business (for example, an American automobile) must be increased.

The following is an interview with a Nashville business executive who has employed workers with diabetes. He was sensitive to the plight of employees with diabetes and other chronic diseases, having worked closely with two individuals who had diabetes, but as a businessman he was also keenly concerned about the necessity to limit health care costs for his company.

Q: What are your considerations regarding health before hiring?

A: My first thought is whether anything would restrict the person from doing the job. In other words, are there demands of the job that the person couldn't perform because of the health condition? I also want to know if there are any potential emergencies that I, as a coworker or boss, might need to respond to.

Q: What has been your experience in hiring workers with diabetes?

A: I've had close experience with two employees. The first is my trusted and valuable assistant who began working with me twenty years ago. The second worker stayed only about two years.

Q: How has the performance of these two workers been?

A: The first employee mentioned has been a valuable teammate. She is very conscientious in managing her diabetes, and it seldom interferes with her work. The second employee was the opposite: absent a lot, couldn't perform on a regular basis, didn't make any positive contributions to the group. It was due to her health. I would not hire her again because of too much absenteeism, too many interruptions.

Q: What is your attitude about absenteeism?

A: Absenteeism affects the ability to use a person in a productive way, especially on a project that has deadlines. Everyone understands that people get sick from time to time, and they are usually sympathetic and understanding, but repeated absenteeism impacts coworkers. Sometimes they have to do more work, and they're not being paid extra for it. If it happens a lot, coworkers resent it, even if it happens for health reasons.

I've had some situations where work could be rescheduled. The Internet makes it possible to get work done from different locations. The employee might feel better that evening and could do the work at home or on the weekend and e-mail it in.

The employee who was absent a lot was terminated after she used up all her sick days and sick leave, all her vacation time, all her long-term disability and family medical leave, and everything. While on long-term disability, she got full salary for a while, then partial salary. She ran through all the benefits the company provided. The benefits lasted a long time and were worth a lot financially. I hope she was appreciative of the extended benefits for several months at no expense to her and at considerable expense to her employer.

From an economic perspective, if you're able to get a group of employees who are healthy and not absent much and don't use health care much, it will save money and increase profitability.

Q: What about health insurance costs?

A: That's an increasing concern for employers. In big business, there's been a definite trend to encourage employees to improve and maintain good health, not only because it helps them to be at work consistently, but because it helps to reduce health care premiums. We do free health screening for employees and provide an 800 number for counseling. My company even pays part of my costs for a membership at an exercise club. Exercise, hopefully, reduces some health problems, and can save money in the long term.

When you have a large pool of people, you have a representative sample of people with chronic disorders like diabetes. In a small business, it might be different.

Q: What would be your attitude if you were running a small business with ten employees, and there were two equally qualified people, but one had diabetes?

A: The majority of jobs are with small businesses. A small business is on a tighter survival line and doesn't have as much flexibility as a big business which has more capital, more reserves, and more ability to absorb unexpected costs. If I were running a small grocery store with just a few employees, I wouldn't hire someone with a chronic illness if I could hire someone healthy with equal abilities. If you have to answer the phone or are a cashier at a retail store, you can't make up that time in the evening.

I would advise someone with diabetes to be employed by a large company with a comprehensive health plan where any potential cost of the condition is shared among a big group of participants in the program. As long as the condition and its needs fit within the norms of actuarial calculation, its cost can be absorbed.

My large company has a policy of accommodating people with health conditions and disabilities of various types. We have special programs like flextime, work from home, and job assignments to fit the abilities of a person. We recognize that these people are an important segment of the population. If we make productive work possible for them, it will result in positive spinoffs for our business, and our company will be recognized as a good and understanding employer.

In 2007, the per capita medical expenditures for people with diabetes were $11,744, approximately 2.3 times higher than average costs for people without diabetes. The cost of diabetes in America was at least $174 billion.[1]

CHAPTER 22

On the Road and In the Air

Jack had driven an eighteen-wheeler since he was eighteen. He had made a good living, supporting his family by working as a commercial truck driver. He had driven to forty-nine states, including Alaska. He'd never had an accident.

Somewhere along the way, he had developed diabetes. He couldn't remember precisely when—possibly during his twenties or thirties. He had gotten sick and gone to an emergency room, where the doctor had told him he'd have to take insulin for the rest of his life. He did what the doctor told him and had always felt fine.

Jack had had an occasional hypoglycemic reaction, but never while driving. When he drove, he had cut back on his insulin dose and let his blood sugar run a little high. He had always carried candy bars in his glove compartment, just in case, but he had never needed one. He didn't smoke or drink. He had taken good care of himself. He had heard tales of guys acting crazy or losing consciousness and going into a coma because of low blood sugar, but it had never happened to him. The idea of an eighteen-wheeler going down the road without a fully aware and competent driver at the wheel was repugnant to him.

During his career as a truck driver, the U.S. Department of Transportation (DOT) required a physical examination and medical certification every two years. One of the questions was "Do you have diabetes?" He always answered no. He knew that if his employer found out that he had diabetes and took insulin, he would lose his job. He feared the urinalysis: sugar would appear in the urine if the blood glucose level had exceeded 170 mg/dl at any time since the previous emptying of the bladder.

Jack's scheme for avoiding glucose in the urine, according to my recollection, went something like this. He scheduled the examination as early in the morning as possible. On the morning of the exam, he took his usual dose of insulin plus a few extra units, then skipped breakfast. Immediately before entering the exam, he emptied his bladder to be certain it didn't contain any urine from an earlier time when his blood sugar might have been higher. Then he drank some water so that when he was given the container for the urine specimen, he could produce an adequate amount for the test. Since he hadn't eaten breakfast, he knew there was a definite risk of low blood sugar during the exam, especially if the doctor was late or the exam took longer than usual. Low blood sugar sometimes produced sweating or nervousness, but somehow Jack always managed to get by. As soon as the exam was completed, he ate a candy bar. He never flunked the exam or was disqualified from his job.

Several years after Jack retired, the Federal Motor Carrier Safety Administration (FMCSA) at the DOT replaced the blanket ban that had prohibited anyone with diabetes who used insulin from driving commercial vehicles in interstate commerce. The FMCSA provided a protocol for case-by-case review to issue exemptions to certain insulin-using diabetic drivers. Congress passed a new transportation bill in 2005, requiring that individuals with insulin-treated diabetes demonstrate stable control of diabetes while taking insulin and fulfill fifty-seven other criteria listed in the September 3, 2003 Federal Register Notice (with two revisions in the November 8, 2005 Federal Register Notice). These requirements included: an annual examination by both a medical examiner and an endocrinologist; written confirmation from the endocrinologist on a quarterly basis regarding the details of glucose monitoring correlated with daily records of actual driving times; the driver's compliance with stringent guidelines to monitor his blood sugar every two to four hours while driving and taking appropriate action to maintain it in the range of 100 mg/dl to 400 mg/dl; and the driver's freedom from severe hypoglycemia within the past five years.

Freedom from severe hypoglycemic reactions in this context means no recurrent (two or more) hypoglycemic reactions within the past five years resulting in loss of consciousness or seizure, requiring the assistance of another person, or resulting in impaired cognitive function that occurred without warning symptoms. For each of these, a period of one year of demonstrated stability was required following the first episode of hypoglycemia.

Aircraft pilots with diabetes are also subject to restrictions, with exemptions for certain individuals who would likely perform safely.

Simon was eighty years old when he sold his airplane and had to give up flying. "I was getting more deaf," he said, "and when I used the radio for conversations with the ground, those fellows on the ground had to keep repeating themselves, and they didn't have time for that."

The airplane was a four-passenger Mooney M20J. Simon's usually impassive face lighted up when he described it. "It looked like a fighter plane. I owned my first one for fifteen years, then the second one for five years."

Flying had aroused Simon's interest when he served just after high school in aviation fire control for the Marine Corps during the Second World War. After the war, he knew he didn't have the time or money to pursue his interest in aviation. He went to college, got married, raised four children, and worked as a construction contractor. At age fifty-five, he obtained his pilot's license, and subsequently he flew almost daily. "Sometimes I would just fly up to Lake Barkley State Park in Kentucky, where they have a fine landing strip," he related. "I would eat lunch at the lodge, maybe fish for a few hours, then fly back to Nashville. Sometimes I would fly to Texas, or even to Arizona."

He particularly enjoyed flying to Midland, Texas, where he would attend the Confederate Air Force Museum (aka the Commemorative Air Force Museum or American Airpower Heritage Museum), which chronicles WWII military aviation. After his wife died, he met a woman who had been a stewardess for American Airlines. She loved flying and often accompanied him until she died also. When asked what he liked about flying, he thought a while and then replied with a trace of a grin, "It gives you a high when you leave the ground."

At age seventy-five, Simon developed type 2 diabetes. He was able to control the condition with pills satisfactorily for the first four years. Then, during a respiratory infection, his blood sugar went up, and insulin treatment was required. The elevated blood sugar persisted even after the infection, so permanent daily insulin treatment was needed.

The Federal Aviation Administration (FAA) has an established policy that permits special medical certification for individuals with insulin-treated diabetes. The certification requires substantial documentation and monitoring. These individuals are eligible only for third-class airman medical certificates, which limits their privileges to that of recreational or private pilots within the airspace of the United States.

Simon was delighted with this policy, but first his diabetes had to be controlled. During a three-month period just after his seventy-ninth birthday, he began insulin regulation. He had weekly visits or telephone calls with both Anne and a dietitian. He learned to count carbohydrates precisely, and began to administer rapid-acting insulin with each meal in the ratio of one unit of insulin for every ten grams of carbohydrates that he ate. He frequently had hypoglycemia, so the ratio was reduced to one unit of insulin for every twenty grams of carbohydrates, then later to one unit for every twenty-five grams of carbohydrates. He checked his blood sugar four times daily, before each meal and at bedtime. Whenever it was between 150 mg/dl and 200 mg/dl, he added one unit of insulin; if between 200 mg/dl and 250 mg/dl, he added two units; and if above 250 mg/dl, he added three units. His precision and attention to detail were meticulous. His fourth daily insulin injection was Lantus, which provided a constant level of insulin for twenty-four hours. He was very sensitive to even tiny changes in insulin dose, but it was finally regulated to result in virtually normal blood sugars at all times of the day and night. None of his brief episodes of hypoglycemia resulted in loss of consciousness or impaired functioning or thinking, and none required assistance or intervention by another party. All this medical information and documentation, plus examination by an ophthalmologist and a treadmill test by a cardiologist, were submitted to the FAA. Finally, a few months before his eightieth birthday, he received the renewal of his airman certification.

Within thirty minutes prior to takeoff, his blood glucose concentration had to be within the 100 mg/dl to 300 mg/dl range. Every hour during flight, and within half an hour prior to landing, he had to measure and document that his blood glucose remained within that range. If it was less than 100 mg/dl, he had to ingest a twenty-gram glucose snack. If it was over 300 mg/dl, he had to land as soon as practicable at the nearest suitable airport. If variables such as adverse weather or turbulence prevented the hourly measurement of his blood sugar concentration, he was instructed to ingest a ten-gram glucose snack. If the conditions requiring his undivided attention to piloting prevented a second consecutive hourly measurement, the regulations indicated that he was to ingest a twenty-gram glucose snack and land as soon as practicable.

Simon had no problems fulfilling these requirements and would still be in the air if his deafness had not progressed.

CHAPTER 23

A Better Life?

Raul didn't have diabetes when he left his home in the Mexican province of Guerrero for the United States. He wanted a better life for himself, his wife, and his four children. Raul was healthy and athletic. He played soccer at least three days per week, and he usually walked almost three hours every day, covering the five miles to and from the factory where he worked. Occasionally he rode a bus, but he had no car. He bought fresh fruits and vegetables on the streets. His wife made tortillas for the family, and grilled meat or fish over an open fire. He says the food he ate in Mexico was more tasty than that in the United States.

Now, four years later, Raul has a job in a factory in Nashville, where he earns considerably more money than he did in Mexico. He owns a car, and his house is bigger and more comfortable. He played soccer for a while, but after a year or so it fizzled out, and now his main sport is billiards. Raul rarely walks now; he loves driving his car. His wife can buy Mexican foods and spices and generally cooks in the same manner as she did in Mexico, but Raul acknowledges that he eats less fresh fruit and vegetables. Much of the meat and chicken he eats here is fried rather than grilled. He enjoys going out to McDonald's and Chinese restaurants. Rarely could he afford this in Mexico. Raul and his family are happy in Nashville.

After living in Nashville for two years, Raul developed thirst and frequent urination and lost about thirty pounds. Diabetes was diagnosed. He was thirty-five years old. Despite his better-paying job, he had no health insurance. He sought care at a clinic staffed largely by volunteer medical professionals. When Raul arrived at the clinic, his blood sugar was 500 mg/dl, and he was started on insulin.

The clinic where Raul was treated is a nonprofit, faith-based family health center that provides care to the uninsured and others who slip through the cracks in the health care system According to a nurse practitioner at the center, about 80 percent of her patients are Latino, many of them are undocumented, and at least a third have diabetes.

The nurse practitioner said, "I've heard many Latinas associate the onset of diabetes with stress, such as the language barrier, fear of being deported, or difficulty finding a job." After the onset of diabetes, despite education and instruction at the clinic, their eating and exercise habits usually did not change much. When she asked these women if they missed home, many expressed a wish to return but acknowledged they had moved to this country for the sake of their children.

Does the nurse practitioner ever get discouraged about the care of these patients? "I have to struggle with that," she replied. "I have to ask myself why am I working in this role. Am I called to succeed, meaning my patients will have their A1c level below 7 percent and be in perfect health, or am I called to help people understand the wholeness of their health, their body, and their soul?"

> Control of financial need and control of health have not always been parallel in transplanted peoples. While their economic status has improved, immigrants of Mexican, Central American, and Asian origin have also developed high rates of type 2 diabetes after moving to the United States. The problem is not limited to immigrants to the United States. Previously undernourished people from the Indian subcontinent have experienced high rates of diabetes after immigrating to England, and refugees from the interior of Africa have had similar experiences after arrival in South Africa. Development of diabetes among immigrant groups who migrate from underdeveloped countries to the West has posed difficult challenges for both patients and their health care providers.
>
> One of the most demanding examples involved black-skinned villagers from famine-stricken Ethiopia whose first encounters with diabetes occurred after they were relocated to Israel.

We had the opportunity to collaborate with Dr. Anat Jaffe, an endocrinologist who directs the diabetes unit at Hillel Yaffe Medical Center in Hadera, Israel. Dr. Jaffe brought an eleven-member team of diabetes educators, consisting of nurses and other health care workers, for a two-week professional development course at Vanderbilt. The team members were all of Ethiopian descent and members of the immigrant

Ethiopian community. They provided us with the details of the following story.

In a typical village in Ethiopia, nobody had diabetes. Nor did they have running water, electricity, or cars. The people were sinewy and lean, and the village elders were tall, dignified individuals who appeared ageless. They worked in the fields all day, and wherever they went, they walked. They shared their simple thatch-roofed huts with their chickens and lean cows.

For meals, they sat cross-legged on homespun straw mats on the floors of their huts. They tore off handfuls of *injera* (a soft, unleavened bread made from a grain called *teff*) to scoop and roll up bites of peppery stew consisting of vegetables, lentils, or dried peas. There was occasionally meat, but it was usually reserved for feast days or holidays—notably Jewish holidays. These people were descendants of the ancient Israelites of the Old Testament, who had lived in Egypt; they had separated from the other tribes, probably after the exodus from Egypt. According to legend, they had migrated southward and settled in northern Ethiopia, where they had remained, largely isolated from the progress of the rest of the world for over three thousand years. They had been independent, successful farmers; those who didn't succumb to diseases like malaria or other parasitic infestations had lived happy, healthy lives.

In the early 1980s, a series of famines struck northern Ethiopia. These people had always concluded their prayers at Passover with the words "Next year in Jerusalem" and had presumed that at some unspecified time in the future they would become reunited with their relatives in Israel. Now it had become an emergent necessity. Leaving their villages, the Ethiopian Jews walked several hundred miles, many of them barefoot, to secret desert refugee tent camps in Sudan.

After several months of international negotiations, they were rescued and flown to Israel by the Israeli Air Force and El Al Airlines. They had never been on airplanes before. Some described the experience as being flown by a giant bird. Within the mere few hours of a plane flight, thousands of rural people, their only possessions being the robes they wore, emerged into a modern, industrialized country—one with computers, office buildings, and cars zooming down highways.

After the initial jubilation of their rescue, cultural and social problems began to emerge. The new immigrants lacked formal education and work skills for a twentieth-century society. Though the children were sent to school and would eventually integrate more easily, the adults usually persisted in their former ways. Instead of owning land and providing food for themselves, they were living in high-rise apartment buildings. They continued to eat their traditional foods when they could obtain them, but Western food, with fewer fresh vegetables and with higher fat content, was gradually introduced into their diet. They did not consider the new types of food obtained in supermarkets healthy. The primitive agricultural methods of the Ethiopian farmers were not in demand on the mechanized Israeli farms. Without daily work, their previously active lifestyle became sedentary. They were watching television and playing cards instead of raising food. Many gained weight, and some began to abuse alcohol or drugs.

The rescue efforts continued from 1984 to 1991. By 2002, eighteen years after the migration began, 17 percent of the estimated 75,000 Ethiopian Israelis had developed diabetes, a condition virtually unknown in this population before. How had they escaped diabetes for centuries, only to become inundated with it in just a few years?

Ethiopians often had terrible control of diabetes at the same time that they seemed to have lost control over their customs, food, and almost every other aspect of their lives. Ethiopian patients with diabetes were considered by well-meaning Israeli physicians to be uncooperative and difficult to treat, and there were mutual misunderstandings and lack of communication.[1] Medical care, particularly for chronic illnesses, had not been part of life in Ethiopia, where it had been felt that if doctors didn't cure, they were worthless. There was skepticism and distrust of modern medicine and Israeli doctors. The treatment of diabetes, with its emphasis on dietary restrictions, daily insulin injections or oral medication use, self-testing of blood sugar, and laboratory tests, was foreign and frustrating.

To help address the problem, Dr. Jaffe organized a program called *Tene Briut*. *Te'ne* means "health" in Amharic, the Ethiopian language. The word signifies a jewel basket, a valuable gift that one should preserve. *Briut* means "health" in Hebrew. The heart of the project was a team of Ethiopian nurses who were engaged in health promotion in settings like immigrant centers, community centers, and clinics. The program provided culturally appropriate education on prevention and treatment of lifestyle-associated chronic illnesses, with particular emphasis on diabetes. For example, one of the project's activities was a series of cooking classes, in which the participants learned to combine Israeli foods with traditional Ethiopian foods.

The increase in diabetes can be seen not only in immigrants to Western countries: it is now occurring with increasing frequency in the developing world. Already there are more people with diabetes in India than in the United States. The increase in the prevalence of type 2 diabetes is closely linked to the upsurge in obesity in countries adopting a Western lifestyle involving decreased physical activity and overconsumption of cheap, high-caloric food. The number of people with diabetes worldwide is projected to increase from 171 million in 2000 to 366 million by 2030, with India, China, and the Western Pacific region at the forefront.[2]

CHAPTER 24

Semper Fi at the Dialysis Center

Fred still answers questions with a sharp "Yes, sir" or "No, sir," accenting the "sir." On his head is a red baseball cap with the emblem of the U.S. Marine Corps—the eagle, globe, and anchor. The same emblem hangs from the mirror in his car, adorns items in his living room and bedroom, and embellishes the blanket that he brings to the dialysis center. He lies under this blanket for four hours every Monday, Wednesday, and Friday morning, napping or watching sports on television while the hemodialysis machine filters the waste products from his blood, a task his kidneys can no longer accomplish.

"After I saw the movie *Iwo Jima*, starring John Wayne, I wanted to be a Marine. Then I saw some Marines in their dress blues at the state fair. I was a kid then, but I was able to live my dream," Fred says proudly. He served in the U.S. Marine Corps for twenty years and retired as gunnery sergeant, E-7, after three tours in Vietnam.

> From age seventeen, the Marine Corps was the only life I knew. I experienced my young adulthood and maturing into a man in the Marine Corps; all my mentors were in the Marine Corps. I liked the regimentation, the discipline, the camaraderie, the esprit de corps, and the sense of belonging to something.
>
> In Vietnam I was a platoon sergeant, usually in charge of sixty-five to seventy men. On my second tour there, I got wounded, but that was my job; that was what I had trained for. I lost a few. I can remember the first man I ever lost in combat; he was my radio operator, from Utica, New York. I'm biased, but I would recommend the military service to anyone trying to find his way.

Fred developed diabetes and high blood pressure at age fifty-eight. "I was thirsty; I couldn't get enough to drink," he recalled. "I was drinking, drinking, drinking, and going to the bathroom. My friend got his meter out of his car, checked my blood sugar, and it was over 300 mg/dl. There had been no diabetes in my family, and I wasn't overweight. The VA attributed my diabetes to Agent Orange. I had been exposed to it in Vietnam; one hill I was on was sprayed several times. It smelled like Clorox when it got wet. My retirement was switched to disability, and now I draw 100 percent disability." (In 2000, the VA added type 2 diabetes to the list of "presumptive diseases associated with herbicide exposure.")

Fred continues, "Two years later, I had a pain hit me; it bent me over. I knew I was having a heart attack. I called the paramedics, who arrived as my wife happened to call. I told the paramedic to answer the phone. My wife thought she had called the wrong number. She rushed over and met me in emergency. I had a heart blockage; I had angioplasty, and they put in a stent. After getting contrast for the arteriogram, my kidneys messed up." (Radiocontrast agents—dyes administered during X-ray studies to outline blood vessels—can occasionally cause sudden decrease in kidney function, sometimes irreversible. Persons with diabetes are more susceptible to this complication.)

"When I found out my kidneys were not working, I was devastated," Fred says. "For a year, I was in the hospital every month; it was just a struggle. I was scared of dialysis then, but I don't want to die. Now it's hard to keep me away from dialysis. I'm sixty-five, I'm enjoying life, I'm living better than I ever did. I have five children, fifteen grandchildren, two great-grandchildren. I'm always busy, always moving. My wife doesn't allow me to dwell in self-pity."

At the dialysis center, Fred is connected to the hemodialysis machine by tubes inserted into the arteriovenous shunt in the left lower arm. Blood flows out of the arterial side into the dialysis device. After it is filtered, the blood returns to the venous side of the shunt. When he bends his arm, which he does repeatedly, an alarm bell rings, signaling obstruction of the blood flow, and a nurse comes in to check the apparatus. She reminds Fred not to bend his arm and then hurries away to attend to her other patients. Fred chews pink bubblegum throughout the procedure.

About three hours into the dialysis, the alarm bell rings again, and the dialysis machine displays a message that his blood pressure has fallen to subnormal levels. "When my blood pressure drops, I just feel dry," he says. "They might lay me back for a while." The nurse makes some adjustments, and his blood pressure returns to normal. Fred indicates that occasionally he feels weak after dialysis and has to sleep at home that afternoon.

During dialysis, Fred elaborates on his life:

> I've been married four times, that's another story. I could write a book on marriages. But my defining moment, it was the Corps. When I retired from the Marine Corps, that was a culture shock. All these civilians didn't seem organized. The only thing I could do was go to school. The GI bill paid me to go to college. I graduated from Tennessee State University, history-geography major. Then I went to work for the VA. I rose up to a nice position, had a desk with my name on it, but I'm still not used to civilian life twenty-seven years after retirement.
>
> My little circle of friends—we play poker. The other night we started at 5 p.m. and didn't stop until 2:30 a.m. We play Texas hold'em and seven- and five-card stud. We all been friends for years. We all tell lies about what we've been doing, you know, in bed. Truth is, none of us are doing nothing—every one of us is on medication. There's not a soul there not taking a ton of medication. We either got diabetes or cancer or are on dialysis machines. Something is wrong with all of us.
>
> Death—once you die, they mourn a few days, and it's over. But sickness, man, it can go on for years. It drains the sap. Diabetes is all about control—everything in moderation. Don't eat three bowls of soup; eat just one bowl. If you're really with it on dialysis, you got to stay away from that saltshaker too.
>
> Nurse Kathleen is my diabetes doctor. She has treated me good, but sometimes she's chewed my ass out. She's my little drill sergeant.

The patient's options when he develops end-stage kidney disease are delimited by the acronym "DDT"—death, dialysis, or transplantation. Medicare insures most patients receiving dialysis; the average expenditure per patient is about $67,000 annually.[1]

CHAPTER 25

Jocks Face Hypoglycemia

"It was a team effort. We had this play, 26-trio, where the tail-back ran right behind myself, the guard, and the tight end. With the three of us, an eight-hundred-pound mass exploded into one poor defensive lineman. We just blew him up and sent him into the backfield. The play could be run on either side, but it was probably more effective on my side. I love to hit. We won because we hit hard," boasted Jack.

I asked Jack to describe how he handled the combination of football and diabetes. He said:

I was diagnosed in fifth grade. When I went to my pediatrician, my blood sugar was over 600 mg/dl, indicating that my pancreas had issues. Once I started taking insulin shots, I gained weight. The whole school knew I was diabetic. I was in that K-12 school since kindergarten. At first, I was the only one with diabetes, but later a girl a class below me got type 1 diabetes also. In the summer, I went to the Tennessee Camp for Diabetic Children, where I met lots of kids with diabetes. I had diabetes for four years before football.

By the eighth grade, my height was 6'7", and I weighed 208 pounds. Then I quit growing vertically, and I started working out in the weight room. My footwork and coordination never developed, so I concentrated on football. By my junior and senior years, I weighed about 315 pounds.

I played both defensive and offensive tackle. I played all the time except for punts and kickoff returns. On offense, I was the strong-side tackle. I liked defense better because you played with more emotion. You just hit the guy in front of you and went for the ball. I was so much bigger than the other guy, I beat him out most of the time. Once I got by him, I had to think, "Where is the ball, is the quarterback passing, is it going to the tailback or up the middle?" It was easy. Most of the time the ball didn't come my way, but when it did, I caused a few fumbles. I recovered a few, and I got a number of sacks.

During practices and games, I purposely kept my blood sugar high. Coach always pushed us. With our coach, winning was just what you did. We worked hard, practiced 2 1/2 or 3 hours after school, and it was challenging at times. It was miserable, but it was good. We took care of what needed to be taken care of. Coach said I was responsible for 75 percent of the gray hairs in his head.

The only thing I did differently from the other players was to check my blood sugar if I felt low. I had enough awareness of hypoglycemia that I could usually feel my blood sugar getting low. They never had to step in and stop me; I would be the one to say I needed to stop and check my blood sugar. The trainers knew the drill, and sometimes they would remind me to check my blood sugar. With my meter close at hand, I could just stop, take off my helmet and glove, and prick my finger. If my blood sugar was below 70 mg/dl, I'd have a little shot of Gatorade, then go back to work.

There would always be a water bottle with some trainer's tape on top to let me know which bottle had the Gatorade. The biggest problem? Every football player preferred Gatorade to water, and they all knew which bottle had the Gatorade. The trainers had an emergency glucagon kit in case I ever actually fell out, but I never needed the glucagon.

If hypoglycemia had been an issue, it would have come up during two-a-days in August. We practiced twice a day when it was 95 degrees and the heat index approaching hell. That's far more strenuous than a game would ever be. I got through two-a-days without an issue.

When asked what he did when his blood sugar was very high, Jack replied that he would usually "run it down if I felt like it" with wind sprints.

I inquired whether he ever had to come out of a game because of suspected low blood sugar. Jack was vague in his response. "Coach never took me out, but he probably wouldn't have noticed it in the intensity of a game. Whenever I came off the field, I would check my blood sugar. Occasionally, I'd take a whole bottle of glucose tablets or a bottle of Gatorade. That would push my blood sugar up to 300 mg/dl, but I'd rather have it 300 than 30. We had enough depth on our team that it didn't matter if I had to stay out for a few minutes. Most guys had to come out for a breather."

Jack recalls an episode during practice when he felt a little goofy due to low blood sugar. He was flattened and almost seriously injured by a massive block from one of his teammates. He had a mild concussion. "I was kinda in a daze that day," he explained. "But a lot of these guys play like they're in a daze all the time."

Many of the Southeastern Conference and other Division I colleges approached Jack about a football scholarship. He began receiving letters of interest from them as early as his freshman year. His father kept them all resulting in a six-inch stack of letters from colleges all over the country. "They could see on game films that I was not inhibited by diabetes," Jack said. "Every college recruiter said they had a boy with diabetes on their team and that they knew how to look after him. They completely reassured my parents that the coaches would treat the fact that I had diabetes with the utmost respect, but parents being parents, they always worry."

They should worry. Every player hits hard in college football.

Bill Talbert, a former captain of the U.S. Davis Cup tennis team, developed type 1 diabetes at age ten, in 1929. In a speech at a diabetes conference at Vanderbilt University in 1975, he related a hypoglycemic episode experienced on the center court of Forest Hills during a championship tennis match. He had won the first two sets handily, then lost the next two sets. It seemed that he had lost his touch. A fellow competitor who had been watching from the sidelines stopped the match, walked to the court, and gave him sugared water to drink. Talbert recovered, winning the set and the match. Everyone wondered what was in the magic potion that he had drunk.

CHAPTER 26

School Fashion

*For the chronically ill, details are all ... and all
this occurs in the context of active lives that are
filled with the same pressures, threats, vagaries,
and exultations that make of normal living such a
"blooming, buzzing confusion."*
—Arthur Kleinman[1]

The prom dress was robin's egg blue, strapless, with a body-hugging white sash emphasizing her waist. "Then it flared out, poofy, and went to the ground," Sally said proudly as she showed me the photographs. She and her mother had driven an hour to shop for it at a bridal and prom store.

A problem arose while dressing for the prom—where to hide her insulin pump. A fourteen-inch clear plastic tube extended from the pump, and the needle at the end of the tube was usually inserted under the skin in the right lower section of her abdomen. She usually wore the pump in her pocket, but there was no pocket in the dress.

"I got the pump when I was a junior in high school," related Sally. "I love my pump. I had all kinds of problems before and was in the hospital every few years for something. With the pump, I cope better. I'm better controlled. I don't have to eat at the same time every day. Before I got the pump, I hated diabetes completely. If I were going out to eat with my friends, I'd have to stop and hold everybody up. I had to check my blood sugar and take my insulin. Now it doesn't take so long. After I check my blood sugar, it takes only pushing a few buttons to give my insulin." Her friends and boyfriend have watched her operate her pump to give insulin doses for meals and snacks. "I wear the pump in my pocket," Sally continued. "I could clip it on my waist, but I have a problem with that. Once I was walking in the crowded hall at school, and a guy came by with a backpack. That backpack caught on the tube and tore the needle out of my stomach."

Medical researchers have tried to devise insulin pumps that could be implanted surgically beneath the skin, where they would be virtually invisible. To date, these efforts have had only limited success. Once this technology is perfected, Sally could fill the reservoir with insulin about once a month and operate the insulin doses with a remote control device. But right before the prom, there was no time to wait on improvements in medical technology. Sally needed a hollow space—or at least a potential space—where her insulin pump could be worn with the dress.

She tucked the pump into the cleavage between her breasts, where it fit perfectly and was snug. The tube was threaded downward, and the needle tip inserted into the usual site in the abdomen. No bulge could be seen anywhere. "I had never worn my pump in the bra before," she said. "I was able to dance, and it never popped out or bothered me. It stayed in place the entire evening. My friends and my boyfriend knew about it; they thought it was funny. When I had to give an insulin dose, I just took it out and pushed the buttons. It didn't bother anybody."

After the prom, she changed into jeans at a friend's house and put the insulin pump back into its familiar home in her pocket. Then she and her friends went to a post-prom breakfast in the park. "It was two or three a.m. when I finally got home," she said.

Fashion is only a part of the problem that high school and college students encounter with diabetes. Issues involving exercise, competing in athletics, self-image, and relationships occur every day.

Rachel, a first-year medical student, reminisces about her experiences with diabetes and her insulin pump during her adolescence:

I think being a teenager on a pump is hard in so many ways, even though it may be best for the diabetes. I played basketball, cross country, and tennis in high school, and had trouble having the pump attached to my body all the time.

I take my pump off when I shower, swim, and do hard exercise like running or playing a sport where my pump is not likely to stay on. I typically keep my pump on for biking, hiking, working out on an elliptical machine, or walking for exercise.

The other awkward situation with an insulin pump occurs at the beach. In high school, I remember wearing my pump to the beach and wearing "tankinis" so that my bathing suit would cover my pump site. During senior spring break at college, I wanted to be able to wear a bikini and get a tan without feeling self-conscious. My nurse practitioner instructed me in the doses of insulin shots I could inject for that week. I went to the beach and actually went off my pump and back to shots for that week. It was much easier than I had expected.

Being an adolescent and young adult on a pump is not only hard due to these logistical considerations, but also because it is hard to have something always attached to your body. One of the reasons I was hesitant to go on a pump as a teenager was its visibility. It seemed a constant reminder to myself that I had diabetes all the time and would always have it. I wanted to forget about it sometimes. Also, the pump caught the attention of many people. Explaining it to everyone seemed almost like wearing a sign on my forehead saying "I am diabetic." Before wearing the pump, only my family and close friends knew about my diabetes. With a pump, it felt like my diabetes couldn't really be my private or personal business anymore.

Another especially hard thing for people with diabetes in high school and college is handling the dating/party/drinking scene. Sometimes they downplay these situations and get drunk, things like that. The psychosocial part is so much harder than how to get your numbers right.

PART IV

Role of the Clinician–Patient Relationship in the Control of Diabetes

The clinician brings medical knowledge to the clinician–patient relationship, dispensing prescriptions and guidance, while the patient is expected to be the agent who carries out these instructions. The clinician–patient partnership is usually satisfying and productive. Most patients benefit from the collaboration and perceive a need for the supervision of a medical manager, whether they accomplish their goals or not.

However, much of the guidance about diabetes control dispensed by the clinician consists of changes to be made in the patient's habits and lifestyle. When a poor outcome indicates a lack of follow-through on these instructions, it is commonly viewed by the clinician as a lack of compliance. Low rates of compliance with recommendations for diet, exercise, taking medications, monitoring blood sugar, and keeping appointments have a major effect on control and outcomes in diabetes. But few patients make deliberate choices not to adhere to their clinicians' advice. A variety of barriers in the patient's life intrude to frustrate the accomplishment of the clinician's directions. These barriers are often beyond the immediate control of either the clinician or the patient.

Many barriers to diabetes control are worse among poor or uneducated people. These include the lack of financial resources to buy medicine and proper food; the lack of transportation to medical appointments; the lack of family and social support; the lack of safe places to walk and of affordable recreational opportunities; the wide availability of cheap, high-calorie foods; and racial and ethnic disparities in health care.

Barriers to diabetes control are not confined to socially disadvantaged persons. Personality barriers (such as indifference or lack of motivation), self-destructive habits (such as cigarette, drug, or alcohol abuse), mental illness (such as unrecognized depression), and low health literacy or numeracy skills are prevalent in all socioeconomic brackets. Underuse of prescribed medication is related not only to cost but to unanswered concerns about necessity and safety.[1]

Finally, barriers are found within the medical care system. Ineffective communication with clinicians and their staff and inadequate patient education confound diabetes control. Among clinicians, clinical inertia often leads to delay of effective control of both blood sugar and blood pressure. *Clinical inertia* is a term that describes the failure of health care providers to initiate or intensify therapy appropriately during clinic visits.[2] Although clinical inertia usually refers to the failure to respond to abnormal laboratory or blood pressure values, we think that the failure to recognize and respond to deep-seated patient concerns is another type of clinical inertia.

What do doctors think about their role in diabetes control? When questioned, many primary care providers felt that diabetes control was more labor-intensive than treating other conditions, and some said that they did not have adequate time or resources to treat their diabetes patients effectively. Some providers thought that the treatment of diabetes was frustrating, since it could not be cured, and that it challenged their sense of effectiveness and self-image. Most said that the successful management of diabetes relied largely on chronic lifestyle changes that they regarded as outside of physician control. In interviews, physicians reported "horrible struggles" with patients because changes in diet and exercise were so difficult to achieve.[3]

These attitudes are not shared by all primary care providers. We conducted in-depth interviews with several primary care physicians in Nashville and the surrounding communities. One conscientious general internist acknowledged the extra time involved and the difficulty in treatment compared with other chronic diseases, but he emphasized that his goal was to persuade each patient to take control of his or her own health. When patients did not adhere to his recommendations for lifestyle change, he sighed nonjudgmentally, "They are where they are."

Most of the primary care physicians whom we interviewed related that the availability of teams that included nurse diabetes educators, nutritionists, exercise instructors, podiatrists, and other specialists was essential. One family practitioner stressed that, in his opinion, each patient with diabetes needed twenty-three hours of instruction, and he tried to refer them to education programs at the hospital or health department in his town. Another family practitioner commented, "I need more time with the diabetic patients. I usually spend twenty to thirty minutes with them, and they get me behind schedule." An internist described the everyday tension about time constraints that exists in a busy office: "The reality is that you're just so busy, and what needs to be done with diabetes is so hard. I won't keep them more than fifteen minutes, even if the blood sugar is high. I will intensify their glucose control if I can do it easily, but if it's hard, I'm not going to take the time to do it."

He elaborated on his assessment of the conflict: "It's easier to walk into an exam room to a patient with a cough and fever, or a patient with hypertension, but a patient with diabetes will take more time. I have mixed emotions about this, because I became a doctor to help people who were sick, and this is someone I could help. But this desire conflicts with the need to move. There is this tension about needing to move and needing to care. In order to care, you have to stop. In most other chronic diseases, it's not a stop, it's just a yield sign. But with diabetes, there's a big red octagon sign. You really have to stop, and it really takes time."

When asked how he addressed the special needs of patients with diabetes, he responded, "I don't think of a patient as just diabetes. I think of him as a person with lots of things that I should address, including all the preventive services, colorectal cancer screening, mammograms, depression. I even have to document that I asked him about fastening his seat belt. Diabetes is rarely the primary focus of my attention. To explain a diet to a patient, I just tell him to eat less. I tell him that it's important, and why it's important, but I don't coerce him."

For an average primary care physician's practice panel of 2,500 patients, it would take an estimated 10.6 hours per working day to deliver all the recommended care for patients with chronic conditions, plus 7.4 hours more to provide all the preventive care proven to be effective. These demands contribute to long waiting times for patients and inadequate quality of care. A growing proportion of patients report that they cannot schedule timely appointments with their physicians, and emergency departments are overflowing with patients who do not have access to primary care. At the same time, primary care physicians are expressing frustration that the knowledge and skills they are expected to master exceed the limits of human capability, and fewer U.S. medical students are choosing careers in primary care (family practice, general internal medicine, and general pediatrics).[4]

With regard to the patients who don't or can't change their behavior and have persistently uncontrolled diabetes, most of the primary care providers acknowledged their frustrations but accepted their limitations. "Early in my career, I would resent patients who didn't comply with my instructions, but with experience I became more accepting," admitted one.

A cardiologist explained how he viewed the situation: "Each patient dances to the music he is hearing." He described one of his patients with diabetes and heart disease who was managing a store in a shopping center.

One day the cardiologist made a purchase at a nearby store, and before leaving the shopping center, he decided to drop by and visit his patient. When he drove up, he saw the patient smoking a cigarette with coworkers outside the store. The cardiologist related that he knew the patient would be terribly embarrassed if his physician saw him smoking, so he ducked his head below the steering wheel and drove by without stopping.

Rita Charon has observed, "The encounter between health professional and patient lies at the heart of medicine. So many pitfalls are possible—the professional might not be smart enough, patient enough, imaginative enough; the patient might not be trusting enough, brave enough, receptive enough. Yet from this inauspicious meeting between two unlike people proceeds whatever healing medicine might provide."[5]

CHAPTER 27

A Fairly Typical Situation

Eddie and his wife and young daughter live on land that has belonged to his wife's family for so many generations they call it their "homeplace." They work in small factories in nearby towns. Eddie's job involves making wooden doors. When business is good, he can earn about eight hours of overtime by working six days each week.

Eddie developed type 1 diabetes when he was a junior in high school. He handles diabetes in a fairly typical way for a twenty-five-year-old man with otherwise good health. Diabetes hasn't yet had a major effect on his daily life. He never misses work, and he rarely has any symptoms related to diabetes or its treatment. His friends and coworkers who know that he has diabetes notice no ill effects. Many don't even know he has it.

Eddie takes his prescribed insulin injections regularly, and he shows up for his appointments every three months at the Vanderbilt Diabetes Center. There he regularly sees a physician, nurse, and dietitian. Over an eighteen-month period, he has had five visits with dietitians who attempted to teach him how to count the grams of carbohydrates in his food. He was always attentive and polite and seemed to understand the material, but he has rarely applied this knowledge to an actual meal. His diet is usually a sausage and biscuit for breakfast, a sandwich and chips for lunch, and a meat and a starch for supper. His high-fat diet with few fresh fruits or vegetables is fairly typical of most of the people he knows.

When his medical team measured his A1c over the past five years, it indicated that his average blood sugar was about 250 mg/dl (normal would be around 100 mg/dl). This is fairly typical for many patients with type 1 diabetes, most who usually feel well and are working regularly. Eddie did have two episodes of DKA, which had resulted in brief hospitalizations. He says he had "intestinal flu" and vomiting, but he had mistakenly omitted his insulin on each occasion.

The Diabetes Control and Complications Trial (DCCT), a landmark ten-year study at multiple medical centers, involved more than a thousand patients with type 1 diabetes. It showed that the typical patient who entered the study felt well and had an average blood sugar of about 250 mg/dl, like Eddie. If the patient just continued with conventional insulin therapy, taking one or two insulin injections daily, this level of control persisted for the next ten years. But as time went on, the patient insidiously developed abnormalities in the eyes, kidneys, and nerves. Only when intensive insulin therapy was used were these complications prevented or slowed down. Intensive therapy consisted of multiple insulin injections daily or the use of an insulin pump, and it required at least four fingerstick blood tests daily. Intensive therapy also involved office visits with a doctor or nurse every month and weekly telephone calls. The patients who used intensive insulin therapy were able to achieve average blood sugar levels significantly lower than those who continued with conventional treatment, and they had significantly less development and progression of the typical long-term complications of diabetes.[1]

The study demonstrated that there was a real gap between what the typical patient with diabetes did and what it really took to achieve adequate control and prevent complications. Eddie is typical of the conventionally treated group in the research study. He seldom tests his blood sugar, so he never takes advantage of the frequent opportunities to correct it when it is high. "I'm just lazy; I forget; I don't have time," he says, but he always promises he will start doing better. At one office visit, he left his glucose monitor in his truck. He was startled when the nurse sent him to the truck to retrieve it. Since he doesn't match his dose of insulin with the carbohydrates that he eats at each meal, he misses the opportunities to prevent his blood sugar from going too high after each meal. Sufficient care of diabetes just takes a lot more effort and attention to detail than Eddie has been able to muster.

So Eddie is a fairly typical guy who leads a fairly typical life and has fairly typical control of diabetes. After ten to fifteen years of this level of control of diabetes, he will probably have typical long-term diabetes complications. His eyes may need laser treatments to prevent blindness. He may need dialysis or a kidney transplant to prevent death from kidney failure. His chance of having a heart attack will be double those of his contemporaries. If he took a more aggressive role in self-management, using the advice of his medical team, he could reduce these risks significantly, but it would take an atypical amount of effort. From his medical team's perspective, Eddie has the barrier of indifference. He appears to be apathetic and ineffective regarding his control of diabetes.

But is the barrier to the achievement of good diabetes control related wholly to Eddie's lack of initiative, or has the clinician–patient relationship been too superficial? Eddie has a more-or-less typical relationship with his medical providers; I am the physician on the medical team. Could at least part of the problem be related to ineffective communication provided by us, the clinicians—or to some other inadequacy in his medical care? Have we failed to recognize something that could motivate him? Have we probed deeply enough? Have we spent enough time with Eddie to understand more than a cursory review of his history and lab work? Could we search more creatively for something that works? Have we cared enough?

From Eddie's perspective, he is already doing a lot to control his diabetes. Is it all his fault?

CHAPTER 28

Non-intensive Care for Diabetes

During his first clinic visit, Michael talked circuitously about his concerns of developing complications of diabetes. He didn't feel ill or have any physical symptoms, but he was terrified. He said he wanted more intensive care. Intensive diabetes treatment aims to produce blood sugar levels as close to normal as possible. This form of therapy requires frequent fingerstick blood sugar monitoring, at least four times daily.

Michael jumped from one topic to another, and it was difficult for me to determine exactly what he hoped to derive from this encounter. He spoke at length of his dissatisfaction with previous doctors. He ignored most of my questions or replied to them tangentially, seldom supplying the information I was seeking. As he spoke, I could feel the tension rising between us. It seemed he wanted to ventilate more than he wanted my advice. I considered that he might derive more benefit from a diabetes support group than from another diabetes specialist. I envisioned Michael going to yet another doctor, and adding the current visit with me to his list of unhelpful medical confrontations.

Michael wasn't doing very well with diabetes. He had not checked his blood sugar for the past month. There was protein in his urine, indicating that diabetes had begun to affect his kidneys. His A1c was 10 percent, indicating that his average blood sugar was about 240 mg/dl, the normal being less than 125 mg/dl.

He had gone to a diabetes clinic at a university hospital in another city, but he insisted he hadn't been helped there. In fact, the experience had been dreadful. "They wanted me to check my blood sugar four times each day, and testing my blood sugar just makes me nervous," he said. It wasn't clear what had upset Michael more—pricking the finger to test the blood sugar or seeing the high results.

Michael worked as an auto mechanic, and he said he couldn't get any work done if he always had to interrupt it to test his blood sugar.

Occasionally, he had low blood sugar that left him weak and listless, unable to work for the rest of the day. Both his parents had died in the past year, and there were other family problems. He was taking an antidepressant medicine, but said it wasn't helping much. His blood pressure was high also, and though two different medications for high blood pressure had been prescribed, he was taking neither. He was restless and his speech was quick, delivered in bursts.

Listening closely, the most frequent complaint I heard was the burden of testing the blood sugar frequently. When he did test, Michael wasn't using the information from the test to calculate his insulin dosage. He just viewed the number and was horrified that it was so high. I concluded that, in his present state of mind, he was not prepared to focus on a set of instructions to lower his blood glucose systematically and safely.

Michael had said he wanted more "intensive care" for diabetes. Perhaps his notion of "intensive care" was that someone would take care of him intensively. Was he looking for a doctor to take care of him, rather than instruction and empowerment to take care of himself?

Conceivably, improvement could be accomplished in a hospital, with nurses testing his blood sugar and administering insulin several times daily, but health insurance wouldn't pay for this type of hospitalization. There were no family members or close friends to help; it was up to Michael. How could I engage him, focus his attention, and win his trust? I was dealing with despair and anger, not merely a disorder of blood glucose. The reason the previous medical advice had failed was the lack of concordance between this patient's needs and his physicians' agenda.

I remembered some advice from a psychologist colleague. She had taught me that patients with a change in their lives go through a spiral of emotional reactions analogous to the stages of grief preceding death. Denial, anger, and sadness are normal responses to abnormal circumstances, and patients can't control their emotions. "Of course you feel that way; it's natural," she reassures patients. Additionally, each medical visit represents a threat of giving up more control—to the illness, to the physician, to the medical establishment.

I was forced to examine my agenda. My underlying concern was the same as what Michael claimed was his—fear of the long-term complications of diabetes—but anguish, not the details of insulin dosage, dominated his agenda. Another formula for adjusting insulin would meet with the same results as previous attempts. "Intensive" insulin therapy was too "tense" for Michael. I had to let go of my agenda, at least temporarily.

Should every patient be compelled to undergo the most modern and intensive treatment? For many years, patients with diabetes had been treated without pricking their fingers to measure the blood sugar, albeit not as effectively as now. I asked Michael how he would feel about continuing treatment for diabetes without being required to test his blood sugar. He stared at me with astonishment, like I had just thrown him an unexpected curveball. Even though he wasn't doing it currently, he had been taught that blood sugar monitoring was one of the essentials of treatment. After he assimilated the shock, he seemed relieved, though apprehensive. He volunteered that he would test his blood sugar at least once daily. Frankly, I was pleasantly surprised by that response. He expressed disappointment that this was not considered "intensive treatment," but he reluctantly acknowledged that his treatment so far had neither fulfilled the definition of intensive treatment nor achieved its potential results. He expressed no disappointment in decreasing the number of insulin injections from four to two daily.

Intensive care isn't for everyone.

Many patients and their physicians have poor agreement on the goals and strategies of diabetes treatment. This suggests that sometimes they fail to work together as a team, or even may be working at cross-purposes to each other.[1]

CHAPTER 29

Driving Under the Influence . . . of Too Much Insulin

When Jason developed diabetes at age seven, his parents took him to the best diabetes specialist in town. This doctor had a convincing bedside manner, and his management of patients with diabetes was regarded with high esteem throughout the community. He told the youngster that if he allowed his blood sugar to be high, he could go blind; at least, that's how Jason remembered it.

Jason has been so afraid of developing blindness from high blood sugar that, ever since childhood, he has repeatedly taken more insulin than he needed, virtually daily. As a result, he has had frequent episodes of confusion or coma due to serious hypoglycemia. He never has any warning symptoms before he blacks out. A perplexing minority of patients like Jason are obsessed with compulsively preventing any elevation of blood sugar, leading to frequent life-threatening episodes of low blood sugar.

Hypoglycemia has been responsible for Jason's multiple auto accidents and even more instances of his being found unconscious in his car at the side of a road. Several years ago, he lost consciousness while driving and sustained a serious head injury, as well as fractures of his left arm and right ankle. He was hospitalized in the intensive care unit at Vanderbilt, where he remained unconscious for several days.

I have been Jason's physician since 1998. After learning of his history, I warned him repeatedly about the dangers of hypoglycemia, especially while driving. I emphasized that he could destroy not only himself but someone else. I hoped that he would respond more to the danger he posed to another, innocent person than he had to his own risk. I knew of an incident where a diabetic patient had lost consciousness due to hypoglycemia, causing a head-on collision. The patient with diabetes had survived, but the driver of the other car had been killed. When I told Jason this story, he listened attentively, but his behavior did not change.

I gave him detailed instructions several times about how to decrease his insulin dose safely, but nothing changed. At every clinic visit, he said that when he tried to reduce the insulin dose, his blood sugar became higher, and then he was afraid he'd go blind, so he always resumed the previous dose.

In November 2003, he was found unconscious in a grocery store parking lot. In May 2004, police found him comatose in his car at roadside with his blood sugar subnormal at 31 mg/dl. In December 2004, while cooking chicken in his kitchen, he lost consciousness due to hypoglycemia. When paramedics arrived, the stove burner was on high, the water had boiled out of the pot, and the chicken was in ashes. In September 2005, he sustained multiple cuts and bruises when he ran into a tree and totaled his car. The frequent dangerous episodes of low blood sugar didn't seem alarming to him. He just accepted them as part of the condition of controlling high blood sugar.

I became progressively horrified about the threat of his injuring someone else in an automobile accident. I thought his repeated episodes of hypoglycemic coma rendered him incompetent to drive and told him so. I familiarized him with MADD, the organization of mothers against drunk drivers. Jason had never married nor had children, and he lived alone. His only relative was his sister, who agreed with me but was powerless to control him or stop him from driving. I threatened to take steps to revoke his driver's license if he didn't decrease his insulin dose.

Finally, I suggested that he seek another source of medical care, since in my opinion he was deriving no benefit from office visits with me. Perhaps another physician would be more influential. He ignored this suggestion also. He said, "You're my doctor." I decided I would not discharge him from my practice or abandon him just because he wouldn't do what I recommended.

If Jason had a communicable disease like diphtheria or syphilis, I would be required to report him to the local health department to protect the health of the community. If I reported a patient with syphilis against his will, even though it was a breach of patient confidence, I would be exempt from a lawsuit. I consulted an attorney to clarify my role as a protector of the community's safety versus the maintenance of the confidentiality of the doctor–patient relationship. I learned that there was no legal requirement that I report my opinion of this patient's incompetence to drive a car to the Department of Motor Vehicles. If I reported him, I had no immunity from a lawsuit regarding breach of patient confidentiality.

Now Jason is fifty-three years old, having "controlled" diabetes for forty-six years. His vision is fine. He drives his car every day. Hypoglycemia resulting from his obsessive habit of taking dangerous excessive doses of insulin has been the dominant factor in his life. In my opinion, the treatment has been far worse than the disease.

Jason has been the most challenging and frustrating patient I have known. I am ashamed to admit that my attitude toward him has ranged from supportive to threatening to sarcastic. I don't think I have been helpful, but he likes and respects me. I wish that he would like me less and follow my medical advice more.

According to studies using a driving simulator, driving performance is significantly disrupted at relatively mild levels of hypoglycemia. Driving off the road, driving fast, and inappropriate braking were the most frequent impairments. Even when subjects were aware of their impaired driving, they often hesitated or waited too long to take corrective action. Individuals who take insulin should not drive without first taking a carbohydrate snack if their blood glucose is below 90 mg/dl, and they should not drive at all when their blood glucose is below 70 mg/dl.[1]

CHAPTER 30

I Had to Sell My Milk Cows

Dairy farming can be profitable, but it's hard work: milking twice a day, no days off, calving, growing hay. In order to deal with these demands, the dairy farmer must be healthy.

Nathan and Elaine had grown up on farms within three miles of one another. They rode the same school bus together for twelve years, were childhood sweethearts, and married as soon as Elaine graduated from high school. Seven generations on each side of the family had made their living farming the fertile Kentucky fields between Nashville and Louisville. They all milked, but their main crop had usually been tobacco. "I milked a cow when I was six years old," said Nathan. "My grandfather lived three miles back over there." He pointed at a nearby hill. "This here was my wife's grandfather's land. He hand-milked and poured it into a can."

Their farm is 117 acres of rolling green pasture. Nathan had won the award for the top milking herd in his county several times. He described his dairy farming operation:

> I kept 60 milk cows which I milked by myself twice a day and
> about 120 heifers for replacement or resale. I was milking so
> many cows, the milk truck from the dairy had to come every
> day, and they don't like to do that. I went off and bought a bigger
> milk tank. The tank was refrigerated and the milk would keep
> so they could come every other day. I had registered Holsteins
> most of the time, but I've always liked the Brown Swiss cow bet-
> ter than anything.
>
> I never sat down much. I got up at 4:30 a.m. and milked
> three hours. I had a small dairy barn with a milking parlor
> where nine or ten cows could eat while they were milked. The
> cows entered the barn on a 12' x 50' concrete floor. I had to get
> behind each cow and push her into the parlor. I milked from the

rear of the cows, not from their sides, as they were packed side by side in the parlor. I did all the labor myself.

Nathan is especially proud of the technique of clipping the cows' tails he had devised. The tails were so short that they didn't get soiled with manure and were not in his way as he milked.

After the morning milking, he would cut hay or harvest crops for winter feed, then milk again at about 4:30 p.m. "My cows grazed in the summer on grass or clover, and I chopped my silage, wheat, hay. In the winter I was working and feeding all the time. It was never over for me. I had expensive cows and artificially inseminated them with the best bulls in the nation. I always kept the baby calves and bought others for replacement or resale. I didn't want to lose a calf. If I was worried about one, I would check it at 10 p.m. before I went to bed, then again at 2 a.m., then again at 4 a.m. After a calf is about two weeks old, it can learn to drink milk from a pail. It was less expensive to buy powdered milk for the calves and sell the cow's milk."

While Nathan milked, Elaine kept the books and ran the business. "I can't do math and she can," he elaborated. They had decided that both of their children would get a college education, which their dairy farming operation supported. Their son had helped with the milking until college, but after graduation he had gotten a higher-paying corporate job in Louisville.

Nathan said he had tried raising beef cattle and couldn't earn a nickel, but he could make dairy farming work. For fifteen years, Nathan never took a vacation. "Elaine and I might go to Nashville or to a dairy convention for a night or two, and my son would milk," he said. When his daughter became ill, she was hospitalized at Vanderbilt for several weeks. One Friday evening, his son came home from college and milked, enabling Nathan to visit his daughter. On the day that she had surgery, Nathan's brother and father and Elaine's brother milked, and Nathan and Elaine had been able to stay in Nashville overnight. Nathan recounted the episode: "My brother is a city man; he left the farm when he was twenty. Elaine's brother is a farmer, but he's a beef farmer; he doesn't know anything about milk cows. But my dad knew how to do it, and they got it done. I was gone only one night."

And then, four years ago, diabetes entered Nathan's life. He was visiting his local physician in a nearby small town for adjustment of his high blood pressure medication. "The doctor snapped his finger and said, 'I know what's wrong with you—it's diabetes. Your mother has it;

your sister has it; your brother has it.' A nurse came in and drew some blood, and I was diagnosed with diabetes."

He took pills for diabetes and felt well for a few years, but when his daughter became ill, everything began to fall apart. Elaine says it was due to stress, because she stayed with her daughter at Vanderbilt Hospital and Nathan had to handle the farm alone. His strength and energy vanished, and sometimes he let his son and father milk in the afternoon. He developed severe thirst and had copious urination day and night. He lost weight rapidly. The local physician prescribed a different pill for diabetes. When this had no effect, he prescribed two different types of pills. When they didn't work, he prescribed a third type of pill to decrease Nathan's blood sugar.

Even with three different types of pills, Nathan's blood sugar remained high, and he felt progressively weak and rundown. The physician increased the dosage of the pills. It made no difference. Elaine said that Nathan was so tired he fell asleep immediately after dinner. "I had always been strong," said Nathan, "short and stocky and strong, but now all I wanted to do was lie on the couch and sleep. I told Elaine 'I'm sick. I can't do it any more.' It got so bad I had to sell my milk cows."

The auction was held at Nathan's farm on a blistering hot Saturday in June. Because of the heat, not as many buyers as expected showed up. The price was not what Nathan had hoped for, but all the milk cows were sold that day.

Even after selling the milk cows, he still couldn't do more than sit on the couch. "I said that I'd just rest and try to get well," but he didn't feel any better. He had no income. Three months after the auction, his doctor mentioned insulin treatment for the first time.

At the time of his first visit to the Vanderbilt Diabetes Center, Nathan's blood sugar was very high. He felt lousy from uncontrolled diabetes. It was obvious he needed insulin. He started on insulin that day and within a few weeks felt much better. He rapidly regained much of his strength and the weight he had lost.

As his new physician, my initial reaction was regret—that he had been treated so ineffectively for so long, until he had become too weak to milk his cows. Why hadn't his local doctor prescribed insulin, or at least referred the patient to someone who could? On insulin therapy, he might have been able to continue dairy farming for many years.

Primary care physicians face many questions and barriers about starting insulin treatment for type 2 diabetes. Some physicians still believe that insulin should be used only as a last resort in patients with type 2 diabetes, after all other available therapies have been tried.[1] In the setting of severely uncontrolled diabetes, with typical symptoms and weight loss, insulin therapy is the treatment of choice and should not be delayed. In many cases, a single daily bedtime injection of insulin, while continuing the pills prescribed earlier, can normalize the fasting blood sugar quickly.[2] Recently published guidelines simplify and encourage the appropriate use of insulin throughout the primary care community, where 90 percent of all patients with type 2 diabetes are treated.[3]

Six weeks later, Nathan's problem had a different focus. He was only fifty-two, and he wondered what he would do with the rest of his life. He knew he could return to work, but he had been a self-employed farmer all his life. He couldn't envision working for someone else or taking a "public" job. Someone had suggested that he apply for disability. "No one in our family has ever taken government help. We just don't believe in that," he said. "Maybe I shouldn't have sold the cows."

When asked why he hadn't hired someone to help with the milking so that he could work shorter hours and occasionally take some time off, Nathan replied, "We've done everything on the farm ourselves; it's a family operation. My mom and dad helped us get our crops in, and we helped them. We've always done it the old-timey way. If you hire somebody, they won't take care of your cows. They won't watch them. You get one infected udder and it may cost you over $1,000. If you don't get them milked out every milking and watch that milk line, they'll get infection. If they get infection in that mammary system, that cow is ruined. You can try; you can give her penicillin or tetracycline. There are four teats on a cow, but once one of them gets infected, you'll never get as much milk out of her. She's good for nothing but beef. The milk company docks you for having a high somatic cell count, so you don't get a good paycheck. Mastitis will put you out of business." In other words, the job wouldn't have been done as well as Nathan had always done it.

When Nathan sold his milk cows at auction, he kept 100 young heifers. He and Elaine thought that if he got well, he could eventually milk again and continue their farming operation. "He just fed them. He didn't milk for over a year," Elaine related. With no income for over a year, money was still going out. Feed costs, especially for corn, were expensive—so much that Nathan planted a field of corn, something he hadn't done for ten years. There were other substantial expenses, particularly for medicine and for health insurance. The savings Nathan and Elaine had been accumulating for a new house were exhausted. He tried milking again for a month but didn't feel well enough.

"I couldn't get out there and push those cows," he said. "Some of them weigh up to 1500 pounds. My dad is seventy-eight; he helped me clean up and sanitize the milkers, but he wasn't strong enough to push them. A cow is stubborn—you have to be strong and used to heavy gates and equipment."

It was costing more to milk than he was making. When he got a good offer, he sold his remaining cows. He learned later that one of the cows he sold broke the three-year-old Kentucky state record for annual milk production. Elaine went back to school and took a job in town as a secretary.

When I visited Nathan and Elaine two years after he had sold his milk cows, he lamented, "If I was able, I'd try to milk again. Dairy farming is good around here now, and corn and soybeans have also made money. I'd like to stay on the farm, but I can't work like I used to."

The economic impact of diabetes includes both the direct costs of medical care and the indirect costs to society of lost productivity and loss of tax revenues. The effects of lost productivity are even more substantial than the direct medical costs of diabetes care.[4]

CHAPTER 31

If Shoes Could Talk

After working fifteen years delivering pizza, Jack could make up to $15 per hour with tips. His tips for a home delivery usually ranged from $1 to $3. He was paid in cash for the pizza and often had to make change. For the coin portion of the change, he would fumble around in his pocket for a while. "One of the tricks of the trade," he acknowledged. "I was hoping that the customer would just say, 'Forget it.'"

Once he made twenty-five deliveries during an eight-hour shift. Some drivers could make even more, because they drove faster, ran red lights, and took more risks. He was instructed always to run to the front door. If the delivery was on the third floor, he would go up the steps as fast as he could. His only reservation about his work was being required to attach the pizza sign to the roof of his car with magnets and straps. If he didn't follow this rule, he would lose his job. The sign might attract new business by advertising, but as Jack said, it also announced that "I'm a delivery driver, and I have at least $20 in cash." Jack described dangerous neighborhoods or apartment complexes where pizza delivery drivers had been robbed or injured. He had been fortunate.

His luck changed abruptly when he was sixty-three years old. While putting on his shoes for work one day, he noticed a vague soreness on the bottom of the left heel. He did not recall any injury to the foot, and there had been no nail in his shoe. He had no idea how it started. He thought he was in good health, and he took no medicine. His wife looked at his heel and said, "Something's oozing out. It looks like an old fashioned boil; it'll come to a head." She got some peroxide and cleaned it up. Then she said, "I think I see a bone there."

When he was examined at the hospital, he couldn't feel the prick of a sharp pin below the middle of the calf on either leg. An unnoticed ulcer on the bottom of the heel had penetrated to the heel bone without Jack feeling anything. A staph infection of the heel bone was diagnosed. By that point, there was nothing that could be done other than amputation of the foot. In order to accomplish removal of the entire foot, including the heel, the amputation was performed just below the knee.

"When the doctor asked, 'Describe the pain. Is it sharp pain? Is it dull pain? Is it nagging pain?' I didn't know. I had lost all feeling in my feet. I didn't know I had diabetes either, before then."

Jack should have known, however. A few years earlier, his physician had obtained routine laboratory tests that had revealed mild elevation of his blood sugar, but Jack had never been informed. Even if the blood sugar levels had been only minimally elevated, the diagnosis of diabetes should have been established and its significance explained to the patient at that time. A therapeutic alliance between the physician and the patient could have been formed, with the expressed aim of controlling this progressive, chronic disease and preventing complications. At the time of the diagnosis, a complete medical evaluation should have been performed, including careful examination of the nerve function and circulation in his feet. This should have been followed by comprehensive diabetes self-management education (DSME), where he would have received instruction in the care and daily inspection of his feet.[1]

The actual sequence of events was probably as follows: Jack had not been aware of a minor injury on the bottom of his foot or of pressure from an unnoticed foreign object in his shoe. (I have found sharp tacks, nails, pebbles, sand, coins, mints, nuts, and paperclips in patients' shoes. Once I found an unopened bottle of fingernail polish that the patient did not feel.) Due to neuropathy and inadequate sensation in the foot, Jack didn't notice the injury or foreign object in his shoe and continued walking on it. An ulcer developed on the sole of the foot. With lack of early detection and with continued pressure, the ulcer penetrated into the deep tissues of the foot. Infection developed there, eventually involving the heel bone.

Detected earlier, the ulcer would have been treated appropriately. A cast or boot would have been prescribed to distribute weight to other areas of the foot when he stood, thus relieving pressure on the ulcer. Adequacy of circulation to the foot would have been checked simply by examining the pulses in the foot or by further tests if necessary. Even if the circulation had been adequate, the foot ulcer probably would have required several months to heal, but amputation could have been prevented.

The surgical site of Jack's amputation healed. During the healing process, he wore a compression stocking to shrink the stump for several weeks to prepare it for a prosthesis. A few months after the amputation, he was fitted with a permanent prosthesis that allowed him to walk.

Every once in a while I have phantom pain in my leg or foot. My brain thinks I still have a foot and toes. Sometimes it's the big toe; it gets to throbbing.

I take off the prosthesis at night. About three months ago, the sock under the prosthesis had blood on it. I had a sore on the stump. It wasn't an ulcer, but it bled when I walked and bore weight on it. It looked like a pone on the nub. [The word *pone*, usually in the compound *cornpone*, means cakes of cornbread fried on a griddle.] I had to take the prosthesis off and air out the bottom of the stump, so I just lay around and watched TV or used a wheelchair. One day I lost a quarter inch of the pone, and eventually it went down to where it was flush and smooth. If it hadn't healed, I would have needed a higher amputation above the knee. Now it's fine.

But Jack isn't able to deliver pizza anymore.

Persons with diabetes should be taught to care for their feet and to choose proper shoes. Sometimes abnormal pressure is caused by poorly fitting shoes. All patients should be screened for neuropathy when diabetes is first diagnosed and at least annually thereafter. The simplest and most sensitive test to detect neuropathy can be done at any clinical examination: A doctor or nurse touches the sole of the foot with the tip of a 10 gram nylon filament similar to fishing line. If the perception of this touch is reduced, the risk of development of a pressure ulcer on the sole of the foot is increased. Special care of feet with reduced sensation is essential to decrease the risk of amputation. Patients with neuropathy should have inspection of their feet at every visit with a health care professional. They should take off their shoes and socks upon entering the examination room and remind the doctor or nurse to examine their feet.

The combination of neuropathy and lower extremity arterial disease (poor circulation) is usually the precursor to amputation in a person with diabetes. People with neuropathy or evidence of increased pressure on the soles of the feet, such as calluses, should use footwear that cushions and redistributes the pressure. Well-fitted walking shoes or athletic shoes are often adequate. People with deformities like hammertoes or bunions may need extra-depth or extra-wide shoes. People with extreme deformities who can't be accommodated with commercial therapeutic footwear may need custom-molded shoes. Therapeutic footwear is an expense covered by Medicare and many health insurance plans.

CHAPTER 32

Everything Is Not Always Due to Diabetes

Erika's main problem was low blood sugar. Her teenage children were terrified by the hypoglycemic reactions, which they couldn't treat in the conventional way they had been taught. They didn't resolve when she drank a glass of juice or ate a few crackers. In fact, sometimes she would chew and swallow twenty glucose tablets before improvement, whereas two or three tablets usually work in most people with diabetes. Erika had had type 1 diabetes for over thirty years, since age ten. In the previous year, she had ended up in the emergency room, unconscious, three times. "I thought something was wrong with my insulin dose—that it needed adjustment," she said. "Everyone, including my family, thought I wasn't doing what I was supposed to do. They accused me of not eating what I should. At work, people were prejudiced against me. They were always wondering if my blood sugar was low. It would take a large amount of food to bring me out of hypoglycemia."

When I first saw Erika, I thought she simply was receiving too much insulin, but there were clues to indicate it wasn't that straightforward. First of all, she also had hypothyroidism. Patients with undiagnosed or undertreated hypothyroidism are more susceptible to low blood sugar.[1] However, Erika had been treated for hypothyroidism for several years, and laboratory tests showed she was receiving the correct dosage of thyroid hormone replacement. Hypothyroidism was not the explanation for her frequent and severe hypoglycemia. She had also had episodes of diarrhea that had been evaluated with many examinations, including x-rays and endoscopies of both the upper and lower parts of the gastrointestinal tract. She had been checked for parasites and infections, and all the tests had been negative.

"All the doctors told me it was due to diabetes—that diabetes could cause just about any symptom," she complained. "In fact, whenever you walk into a doctor's office, the first thing they tell you is that whatever is wrong is due to diabetes. I think there's prejudice against people with diabetes, even among doctors. If you didn't have diabetes, the doctor would be open-minded and consider other alternatives."

The breakthrough in diagnosis occurred because of her astute gynecologist. Erika had had a routine test called bone densitometry, which gynecologists perform to detect the early stages of osteoporosis. The results showed a severe deficiency of calcium in her bones, but she was only forty-four and had not yet entered menopause. "My gynecologist told me that I should be checked to see why I wasn't absorbing calcium," Erika related. "When my doctors continued to blame everything on diabetes, my gynecologist insisted that there was definitely something wrong that hadn't been discovered yet."

Finally, Erika had a blood test for celiac disease. It proved to be positive, and the diagnosis was confirmed by a biopsy of her small intestine. She had malabsorption of fat, protein, carbohydrates, vitamins, and minerals, all of which passed through her intestine unabsorbed and caused the diarrhea.

Celiac disease is a condition in which the immune system responds abnormally to a protein called gluten, causing damage to the lining of the small intestine. It is a treatable condition, but the treatment consists of the lifelong elimination of gluten from the diet, which can be expensive and inconvenient. "Gluten is everywhere," said Erika. "It's found in wheat, rye, barley, and many prepared foods, and it's hidden in additives we use all the time. My gastroenterologist suggested I contact a retired physician who had celiac disease himself. The retired doctor met me at Wild Oats, a grocery that specializes in natural foods, and walked me through the store pointing out what to buy and what to avoid. Rice flour, soybean flour, and potato flour don't contain gluten. I learned I could mix three flours and make bread at home in my food processor. You can buy frozen or refrigerated gluten-free bread, but it's nasty."

Hidden gluten can be found in foods such as cold cuts, soups, hard candies, soy sauce, many low-fat and non-fat products, starches, malts, and even licorice, ice cream, and jelly beans. Gluten may also be used as a binder in some pharmaceutical products. Strict gluten avoidance is recommended since even small amounts can aggravate the disease. Corn, rice, potatoes, buckwheat, legumes, nuts, and seeds are safe.[2]

Erika felt better within weeks of eliminating gluten-containing foods. Now, a few years later, she has gained some weight and has much less frequent hypoglycemia. When she does have low blood sugar, it responds to a small snack or just a few glucose tablets. "I feel pretty good now," she related proudly, "and I'm less tense and irritable."

The combination of diabetes and celiac disease can be difficult to reconcile, since many of the gluten-free food products are high in carbohydrate content. Erika attended several meetings of the Celiac Association of Middle Tennessee:

> Very few people at the Celiac Association also had diabetes. Most of the people there wanted sweets, cakes, and cookies. Mostly they talked about bread-making and sweets. It was ironic for me. I knew better than to follow their recipes. I didn't fit with the usual diabetics and I didn't fit with the people at the Celiac Association, since I had both.
>
> We like to eat in restaurants, but it's very difficult to avoid gluten there. If I ask for a salad without croutons, sometimes the salad still arrives with croutons. The waiter offers to have the croutons removed, but I know that there are crumbs which have contaminated the rest of the salad, so they have to prepare a brand new salad for me. I have to avoid most Asian restaurants because wheat is in soy sauce. We do know of three restaurants in Nashville which have gluten-free menus. One is P. F. Chang's China Bistro, a national chain.
>
> I can eat a few crackers now and not have any symptoms, but the celiac disease would be active, and I would have malabsorption even if I didn't feel sick. My antibody tests would go back up, and my risk for cancer would increase.

Erika is adamant that "everything that happens to someone with diabetes is not always due to diabetes. People with diabetes are like everyone else. We're all different. Doctors should be unbiased in evaluating us."

Though celiac disease affects only about 0.5 percent to 1 percent of all Americans, about 5 percent of persons with type 1 diabetes will develop it. All children with type 1 diabetes should be screened for celiac disease.

The cause of celiac disease was discovered by a Dutch pediatrician who noted that the symptoms of his patients lessened when bread was unavailable during the Second World War, and that their symptoms resumed when bread became available again after the war.

CHAPTER 33

Playing the Numbers

Ken loves numbers. He's a mechanical engineer—a precise, detail-oriented person. "I was fascinated by math since I was a little kid," he said. "In elementary school, I would go through the statistics in the newspaper every day, looking at batting averages and team records. It was always fun for me to take a real-world situation and put a mathematical formula on it." He doesn't remember life without diabetes, which he developed at age three, forty-one years ago.

On the other hand, Ben, a hard-driving salesman the same age as Ken, has a different mindset. Ben explained, "I'm a word man, not a numbers man. I've always been allergic to math. Put a math textbook in front of me and I break out in a rash. I always tell my kids, 'If you need help in English, social studies, history, science, come to me, but if you need help in math, go to your mother.' When I got diabetes, figuring out servings and carbs was always just too much trouble for me."

I asked Ken, the mechanical engineer, how he uses his analytical and mechanical background in managing diabetes. "I make Excel spreadsheets to analyze my blood sugar data. I record the date, the time, the blood sugar, any carbs eaten, and any insulin dose given. I want to see what is actually happening, not just go by the way I feel. I put the blood sugar numbers in categories of less than 70, 70–100, 100–150, 150–200, 200–250, and more than 250 mg/dl. Then I break it down by different times of day: breakfast, mid-morning, lunch, mid-afternoon, dinner, evening, bedtime, and night. The more data you have, the more helpful it will be. I can look at a one-week period of time, a thirty-day period, or any time period I choose. It's a lot to keep up with; it takes time. During my lunch hour, I eat at my desk and update my spreadsheet. I usually e-mail the spreadsheet to Kathleen, then talk to her about what needs to be done."

Ben, the salesman, followed a different road to diabetes control:

I grew up fighting, in a tough neighborhood. In high school, I was second in the state wrestling tournament, and I got a wrestling scholarship. Wrestling got me a free education. If you want me to take somebody down, I can probably do it, but if you want me to count, you're barking up the wrong tree.

I was a professional wrestler for seven years. My gimmick was "260 pounds of twisted steel and sex appeal." I was always the "heel"—the bad guy that the crowd hates. I was never the "babyface." The babyface would get in the ring and start taking his robe off, and I'd jump on him and start beating on him. You're not supposed to start until the bell rings, but I was the bad guy. I brought a lot of comedy into the wrestling match. "Make them love you or make them hate you," I'd say, "but don't let them ignore you."

We produced several TV shows for the pay-for-view market. The biggest show I did, live in front of a TV audience of 11 million people, was at the annual Sturgis Motorcycle Rally, Sturgis, South Dakota. It's the biggest biker rally in the world. In the middle of nowhere, they're drinking and partying all day; there are probably 100,000 bikers in the audience. They're all crowded around the wrestling ring, sitting on bikes. By the time the show starts, around dusk, you got a fired-up crowd. When the heel comes into the ring, you hear all the motorcycles revving. When somebody punched me, they cheered.

Now I'm in an executive sales position. Here's the way I look at it: Wouldn't it be a better use of my time if I were talking to clients rather than crunching numbers? There are people who serve that role admirably and do it well, and they like to do it; I'm just not one of them. Rather than get frustrated and have my diabetes unmanageable, the smart thing was to figure out a way to make it easier for me to manage it.

When Ben arrived at the Vanderbilt Diabetes Center, his A1c was 12.2 percent, indicating an average blood sugar above 275 mg/dl, far out of control. His problem with numbers was recognized, and he was given tools to deal with it: a simple book helped him count the carbohydrates in his meals, and a hand-sized wheel showed him how much insulin to take. "I got myself educated about it," he said. "To use the wheel, I test my blood sugar, enter how many carbs I'm going to eat, then turn the wheel. It tells me what the insulin dose is, I take it and go on my way. I don't have to sit there and put a pencil to it." At his most recent clinic visit, his A1c had decreased to 6.8 percent—a marked improvement.

"I really did turn my diabetes around," Ben said. "I'm your typical immediate- gratification guy. I don't have a lot of patience, I'm high dominance, I'm the perfect sales profile. That means my profile for managing diabetes is exactly the opposite of what it should be."

I asked Ben what constitutes the right profile for managing diabetes. "Somebody who is detail-oriented," he answered. "Somebody who can patiently take the time to figure out what to do. I need the program that any dummy can do."

Ken, the mechanical engineer, fits Ben's profile of the right person to manage diabetes. As we ate barbecue sandwiches, baked beans, and slaw for lunch, I asked Ken how he would handle his insulin for that meal. "I estimate 105 grams of carbohydrate in this meal," said Ken. "I figure sixty grams in the beans, counting the sauce. The sauce doesn't seem sweet, but it has some sugar in it. The bread I estimate about thirty grams. I add the equivalent of about fifteen grams because it's also a high protein meal which needs some compensation for me. Based on what I have learned from my spreadsheets, I have programmed my insulin pump to give me one unit for every thirteen grams of carbohydrate I eat."

He added, "Curiously, last weekend I had a conflict with my teenage daughter. The stress made my blood sugar high for two days afterward. The spreadsheet couldn't have predicted that."

Recently researchers have determined that many patients with diabetes have difficulty using numbers in daily life. Patients had particular difficulties calculating carbohydrates from nutrition labels and determining insulin doses based on insulin-to-carbohydrate ratios. Although there is a correlation between print literacy and math skills, many patients have adequate print literacy but are still unable to use math appropriately. Strategies and tools to help with numbers-related self-management tasks are being developed and tested.[1]

CHAPTER 34

The Doctor Was Hoodwinked

When I first met Melanie, she was a twenty-five-year-old single nurse who worked the night shift at the hospital. She had developed type 1 diabetes four years earlier while in nursing school. She was experiencing hypoglycemia frequently, especially at night, when she worked. She checked her blood sugar ten times daily, understood her insulin treatment regimen perfectly, counted carbohydrates precisely, and reported that she administered her insulin doses exactly as prescribed.

During one clinic visit, she became confused while we were talking. I checked her blood sugar, found it to be low, and gave her six glucose tablets over the next thirty minutes, until her blood sugar increased from 40 mg/dl (very low) to 70 mg/dl (normal) and her mental status gradually cleared. Review of the log on her insulin pump that day revealed that she had given herself insulin doses slightly more frequently than recommended. I explained and corrected her errors.

Twice, her coworkers at the hospital brought her to the emergency room because she had had a convulsive seizure while working. On each occasion, the cause of the seizure was very low blood sugar. She continued to ask me for help in preventing hypoglycemia. I recommended that she decrease her insulin dose, and she understood and agreed, but the incidents of low blood sugar persisted. I couldn't figure out why she had so many episodes of hypoglycemia. I was baffled.

Finally, I learned the explanation. After a seizure at home, an ambulance was called and transported her to the emergency room. She told the doctors there that night that she had been severely depressed, and that all of her hypoglycemic reactions and seizures had been deliberate attempts to kill herself. She had overdosed with insulin at least fifty times. She explained:

You feel bad. You feel that nobody wants you. All these negative feelings circle in your head 24/7. When I got these negative
thoughts, I would say to myself, "What do you have to live for?"
These ideas became foremost in my mind first thing in the
morning and followed me all day. When I got into that mindset,
I was serious about killing myself. I knew depression was a
treatable illness, but I didn't want to be burdened with taking
any more medicines.

I never told anyone I was depressed. I never told a doctor.
I kept it to myself. I overdosed once at my mom's house. Mom
thought it was just low blood sugar, but it was a suicidal act.

During her seizures, Melanie would lose consciousness, have vio-
lent jerking movements, bite her tongue, and urinate on herself. She
would usually awaken on the floor after several hours, and once she
fractured her scapula (shoulder bone) when she fell.

When I woke up after a seizure, I'd be pissed that I didn't
complete what I tried to do. It made me even more depressed,
because I couldn't even kill myself right.

I had great control of diabetes for the first few years until
depression kicked in. Maybe diabetes had a chemical effect on
my brain.

When I checked into the hospital, I was looking for some
help. If they can treat diabetes, they can treat depression. It's
scary when you meet someone who's getting tired of trying to
kill herself. That's how I was.

Melanie had been sexually molested at the age of six and had reported some depression since then. "Things that happened earlier in
my life came back to haunt me. Suicide had been in my mind since
early in [my] life," she said. She had twice been hospitalized for depression voluntarily at another hospital but hadn't told us. A cousin
had committed suicide as a young woman. Her mother, a cancer sur-
vivor, had been taking antidepressant medication. "The depression is
with you all the time," Melanie said. "Occasionally I would drink some
alcohol to get a euphoric feeling—to make me feel good and not think
about the depression."

I asked Melanie if there were any pleasurable sensations from low
blood sugar. "Yes," she replied. "Low blood sugar was like a drug to

me. I would get a temporary feeling of euphoria. I knew it was dangerous, but it made me want to do it more. It was a high—then I'd pass
out. I was depressed, but at the same time I was addicted to low blood
sugar, because it gave me that euphoric feeling every time. If you were
depressed and wanted to kill yourself, you could feel good before you
died. I wanted that happiness before my end."

In response to my inquiry about why she so frequently chose to
overdose with insulin while working at the hospital, she replied, "I
didn't care. I took care of my patients first; everything was fine for
them. I never put anyone else in danger. I'd just get all these negative
thoughts. Suicide is a selfish act; you're only thinking about yourself."

After her first two psychiatric hospitalizations, Melanie stopped
the prescribed antidepressant medications. "Finally, I took the medications and they helped," Melanie said. "I trusted those doctors at the
last hospitalization. Now I'm doing a lot better, and I don't overdose
any more."

Chronic illness, including diabetes, can be involved in the development
of depression. Up to 15 percent of patients with type 1 or type 2 diabetes
meet the official diagnostic criteria for depression.[1] Depression is
frequently underrecognized and undertreated in those with diabetes.
Only 30 percent of patients with depression and diabetes receive
adequate antidepressant treatment.[2] Fortunately, depression among
people with diabetes is just as treatable as it is in any other population.

Contrived hypoglycemia caused by insulin misuse can be difficult to
recognize, because physicians rarely suspect that their patients would
deliberately mislead them or fabricate such a serious illness. Insulin-
dependent diabetes mellitus has been described as a "manipulator's
delight."[3]

CHAPTER 35

A Glimpse of Longevity

Dr. Smithson had competed as a hammer thrower on his college track team. The sport requires an athlete to maintain a position of core strength, spinning in three or four complete turns before propelling a sixteen-pound steel ball through the air. Dr. Smithson's core strength would be tested again by subsequent life events: Years later, as a pathologist, he was involved in research studying patients who had died of AIDS. During a routine autopsy of an AIDS victim, with one slip of his scalpel, he suddenly became infected by HIV. He went from doctor to patient at a time when there was no cure or effective treatment.

He felt strongly that he should control the HIV infection before it progressed to the point of causing the symptoms of AIDS. During the next five years, he took whatever anti-HIV drugs were available, always with the risk of severe side effects or the emergence of resistance that would render the drug ineffective. He and his family thought he was doomed.

Finally, in 1995, saquinavir, the first protease inhibitor, was released, followed shortly thereafter by more potent drugs. Dr. Smithson was elated: "As a patient—as a human stalked by HIV—I feel the grateful joy that I might live. Just four years ago, AIDS hovered like an endless storm, with effective treatments too far off on an overcast horizon to offer hope. HIV meant despair, life without a future, certain premature death. But now, almost incomprehensibly, we're being given a glimpse of longevity. We have reached a new era when HIV may be managed like a chronic disease, like diabetes."

His regimen called for taking thirty-two pills every day. The success of the antiviral drug "cocktail" required a rigidly precise schedule. Some of the five antiviral drugs taken daily had to be taken with food, others on an empty stomach. Colleagues watched as he interrupted his busy work schedule to take multiple pills of different colors, sometimes followed by a sandwich that he had prepared earlier. At least one dose, with a snack, was required in the middle of the night, but he gladly persevered because he felt well, and his laboratory tests showed that the HIV was controlled. In addition, he was in excellent physical shape from his years of track and field and from his subsequent fitness regimen.

While the combinations of antiviral drugs cause profound and sustained suppression of the HIV and prolong life in patients with HIV infections, peculiar effects on body chemistry occur. Within a few months of the initiation of treatment with a protease inhibitor, resistance to insulin can be demonstrated. Insulin resistance is a pre-diabetic condition. If the body cannot effectively compensate for insulin resistance and overcome it, diabetes will result. Insulin resistance is frequently accompanied by changes in blood cholesterol and triglycerides, which predispose to coronary heart disease.[1]

Dr. Smithson and his physicians were aware of his abnormal lipids, but since there had been neither coronary heart disease nor diabetes in his family, and he was so lean and active, they had not been alarmed. But about four years after he began taking protease inhibitors, mild elevation of the blood sugar—indicating diabetes—was noted.

Kathleen was the first member of our medical team to encounter Dr. Smithson: "An endocrinologist colleague asked me informally if I would be willing to counsel a physician friend of his who had been diagnosed recently with HIV drug-induced type 2 diabetes. I met with Dr. Smithson in my office, taught him to test his blood sugar, discussed blood sugar goals, and recommended yet another drug to his extensive list of medications—metformin, a pill that lowers the blood sugar. In order to avoid gastrointestinal side effects, this drug is customarily started at a low dose and increased gradually over several weeks. When I talked to Dr. Smithson a few days later, he reported terrible gastrointestinal symptoms. He told me that he had increased the dose of metformin to the maximum dose in three days rather than the usual four weeks! He said he was well accustomed to tolerating drug side effects, and these were merely a nuisance to him. I realized that he would be as proactive about caring for his diabetes as he was with his HIV."

Five years after starting protease inhibitor therapy, Dr. Smithson sustained a heart attack and required several days of intensive treatment in the coronary care unit. Subsequently, two more medications were added, one to control his cholesterol and another to control triglyceride levels. He initiated tight restrictions to his already spartan diet in attempts to control his diabetes and lipid levels. Three years later, he appeared undernourished. He weighed only 120 pounds—fifty pounds less than his weight as a hammer thrower. He made the decision to initiate treatment with insulin.

Dr. Smithson is doing well currently. Dedicated to the study of pathology, he continues to work long and productive hours, consults with other pathologists about microscopic abnormalities in biopsies or autopsies, and writes papers about his research. His HIV is asymptomatic and well controlled by his cocktail of antiviral drugs. His diabetes and lipid abnormalities are similarly well controlled. "The guiding principles now in selection of anti-HIV drugs are influenced as much by their effects on insulin resistance as by their effects on the HIV virus," he said.

Kathleen commented, "Dr. Smithson always expressed great appreciation for my care. This was ironic, since he actually dictated most of his own diabetes care with minimal input from me."

Occasionally the clinician–patient relationship is easy, but all patients—even proactive ones—benefit from support.

CHAPTER 36

Different Paths to the Same Destination

Anne reflects on working with two patients with widely different personal resources and her lack of success with both.

Thomas is a middle-aged man who has worked in the janitorial department of almost every business in Nashville. His education has been limited. He rides the bus to attend his appointments. He lives alone and does the best he can to care for himself. Often he just can't remember to take his medications, or he runs out of medicine and doesn't take it for long periods. Although sometimes he has insurance to pay for the medications, the complexities of accessing the insurance or the refill procedures at the pharmacy baffle him. In addition to diabetes, he has severe high blood pressure and other medical problems. All in all, he has about fifteen different prescriptions. He does manage to take some of these medications some of the time and to check his blood sugar level most days.

Thomas has progressive kidney disease and will require dialysis or a kidney transplant within a few years. He is at very high risk for a stroke. He faces overwhelming intrinsic barriers that he cannot overcome. I often contemplate concurrently the fates of Thomas and another patient, Nancy.

Nancy has all the resources that Thomas does not—support from a loving husband and family, a rich network of friends, a college education, excellent health insurance, substantial retirement income, and a dependable car. She lives within walking distance of grocery stores and three different health club facilities. She is a retired real estate broker. Former coworkers say that they could always count on Nancy to plan gatherings, outings, and birthday parties.

For Nancy, her bridge dates take priority over her health care appointments. Her luncheons are more important than her medications. Shopping for dresses for her granddaughter is more important than stopping by the pharmacy to pick up blood glucose test strips. She makes conscious decisions to ignore health care advice and goes through life with a garden party attitude. She eats what she wants when she wants. She'd like to be in a smaller dress size for the sake of her appearance, but it isn't worth the effort it would take.

Recently, I became alarmed, because Nancy's urine protein excretion had tripled over the past year. This indicated progression of diabetic kidney disease. I called her to discuss this laboratory result and found that she had stopped taking her medication for this problem six months ago. When I asked why, she replied that she felt just fine and decided that she didn't need it any more. For the past fifteen years, her blood sugar levels have always been in the range indicative of high risk for complications, and we have talked at every appointment about the risks of kidney failure, blindness, and all the other frightening things that most people with diabetes work so hard to avoid. When I ask her pointedly why she is not concerned about these dangers that are so worrisome to me and most of my other patients, she replies, "I'm enjoying life, and when my time comes, it will come. I don't want to worry about those things now." We've even discussed my vision of her future: after a stroke, in a wheelchair, unable to speak, unable to do the things she so enjoys, having to be cared for by others. She asked, "Do any of your other patients act as badly as I do?" Then she laughed as she hurried out the door, late to meet a friend for lunch.

Nancy certainly has the right to choose not to deal with her diabetes. Ultimately, decisions about how to care for oneself rest with the individual patient. But the disparity between the two patients bothers me. Thomas probably would not be facing dialysis soon if he had even a few of Nancy's resources. If he had just a shred of a support system, we could do more to help him, and he could do more to help himself. There is irony in the fact that both Thomas and Nancy are on different paths to the same complications. For Thomas, it's because even the best care he can provide for himself isn't enough, and for Nancy, it's because she doesn't care enough to take advantage of what's provided.

When a patient ignores diabetes, it often means that she is "in denial," meaning that deep in her heart she has never accepted the fact that she has diabetes. Denial can persist for years, with destructive consequences.

Some of the most difficult patients deny that they're in denial. Sometimes a health care provider has contributed to the problem by minimizing its importance, telling a patient that she has only "a touch of sugar" instead of diabetes. Another health care provider may use such severe scare tactics that the patient feels hopeless regarding the management of her disease. It's difficult to walk the narrow line between instilling serious concern in the patient and giving reassurance.

CONCLUSION

Prevention—the Best Method of Control

Prevention of type 1 diabetes is being studied extensively, with a focus on the immunological abnormalities that lead to the destruction of pancreatic islet cells. Therapies are being tested that may delay or prevent the onset of type 1 diabetes in susceptible individuals. Other researchers are studying interventions to preserve insulin-producing cells in people recently diagnosed with type 1 diabetes.

A recent study employing stem cell transplantation in a small number of patients with newly diagnosed type 1 diabetes showed remissions of diabetes and independence from insulin treatment in some patients for up to three years. There was clear evidence of improved islet cell function in the study participants. If the risks of adverse effects of this therapy can be overcome, randomized controlled trials will be necessary to determine the safety and effectiveness of this type of treatment in reversing type 1 diabetes.[1]

While the prevention of type 1 diabetes is benefiting from targeted research, the worldwide epidemic of type 2 diabetes is a critical public health problem. The number of people with type 2 diabetes has increased from 35 million in 1983 to approximately 225 million.[2] Overnutrition and a more sedentary existence now result in 1.6 million new cases per year in the United States. Many of these people will never achieve and sustain normalization of blood sugar. They are at risk for serious complications; therefore, intensive effort should be devoted to prevention.

Prevention of type 2 diabetes is related to obesity and to lifestyle measures. Most current preventive efforts are aimed at the most susceptible—those who are already exhibiting the early blood chemical abnormalities that precede diabetes—although many feel that they should be aimed at the entire population. These abnormalities are called *impaired fasting glucose* and *impaired glucose tolerance*. Impaired fasting glucose and impaired glucose tolerance represent intermediate states between normal blood glucose levels and diabetes. Since the majority of people with these conditions eventually develop diabetes, impaired fasting glucose and impaired glucose tolerance are called *pre-diabetes*. Approximately forty million people in the United States have pre-diabetes—almost twice the number of those who have overt diabetes.

Screening for pre-diabetes should be aimed at those with the greatest risk for the development of diabetes: individuals who have a parent, grandparent, brother, or sister with diabetes; those whose age is over forty-five; those who are overweight; women with a history of gestational diabetes; Hispanic ethnicity, and African American, Asian American, and Native American racial groups.

Lifestyle modification emphasizing modest weight loss and moderate intensity physical activity (about thirty minutes daily) is the treatment of choice for persons with pre-diabetes. However, it is often very difficult to sustain.

The Diabetes Prevention Program, involving 3,234 persons at increased risk of diabetes at twenty-seven sites in the United States and Canada, showed that weight loss and physical activity decreased the incidence of diabetes within three years by more than 50 percent.[3] Achievement of these goals required extensive effort from well-trained staff, entailing considerable expense. Studies in China, Finland, and India have shown similar results.[4]

The authors have a shared personal experience with diabetes prevention. Jamie, our invaluable administrative assistant for several years, knew how to navigate the infrastructure of administrative assistants throughout the medical center to make things happen. We relied on Jamie, and she kept a watchful eye on each of us.

At the same time, we tried to keep a watchful eye on Jamie. We witnessed her daily struggles to cope with her role as a single mother and her battles with smoking and progressive weight gain. As soon as Jamie arrived at the office every morning, she brewed coffee for us, and she kept a fresh pot at her desk all day. "I was putting up to four small creamers in my coffee," she revealed. "They each have fifteen calories, so I had sixty calories per cup, and I was drinking a pot of coffee at work daily."

By the time she was forty-four, she had gained from her normal weight of 150 pounds to 192 pounds. Her primary care physician found her fasting blood sugar to be borderline elevated, indicating pre-diabetes. It was not high enough to indicate diabetes definitively, but too high to be considered normal. "I was awfully concerned about the abnormal blood glucose," she said. "I knew this was serious business, because my father had died of the long-term complications of diabetes."

Jamie had been assisting us in our daily efforts to treat patients with diabetes, our clinical research to determine better methods of treatment, and our educational programs for new physicians and nurses. She had transmitted our telephone messages to patients with diabetes and had been instrumental in developing an e-mail system for patients to communicate with us. Now she was on the patient side of the clinical relationship.

Jamie's primary care physician recommended that she see Anne for instruction in lifestyle changes to prevent progression to diabetes. Anne counseled her about pre-diabetes and referred her to a dietitian for further assistance in losing weight. The dietitian recalled, "From talking to Jamie, I got the sense she was not going to be someone who would be a regimented dieter. Driven by stressful situations, she overate."

Regimented she was not. She lived in an ocean of stressful situations, and she reacted with binge eating. Whenever she tried to stop smoking, she replaced cigarettes with more food. We worried and discussed how we could support her. In the end, we knew it would be up to her.

Within a year, she had lost ten pounds, but still couldn't fit exercise into her schedule or stop smoking. Shortly after I interviewed her for this book, she started regular exercise. It certainly was not due to anything I said. It must have just been the right time. Now she pedals a stationary bicycle at home for thirty minutes every morning. She has lost twenty pounds, so she is halfway to her weight goal, and she has stopped smoking. Her blood sugar levels are normal. Though she has a formidable risk of developing type 2 diabetes, so far she has confirmed that she can prevent it.

The stories in this book illustrate that people with diabetes must work hard to achieve control. But the best method of diabetes control is to prevent it, even if one must work as hard as Jamie. We have made no effort to sugarcoat the seriousness of diabetes. Yet there are strong reasons for hope that scientific research and technological progress have the capacity to eliminate diabetes eventually. The technological advances that have already been achieved, such as insulin pumps and continuous glucose sensors, can command the full attention of both patients and clinicians, outshining all the other elements of control illustrated in this book. But control of diabetes has always been more than control of blood sugar. The lives of our patients and the stories of their living with diabetes depend on individual patient responsibility, family support, the social situation, and the patient–clinician relationship, even with continued scientific progress.

Acknowledgments

Writing this book was fun, but it would not have been accomplished without the help of many people.

After reading a book written by my fellow endocrinologist Clifton Meador about patients that his medical training had not prepared him to manage, I mentioned to him that, in the lives of all my patients with diabetes, there were important elements that interacted in a critical manner with their illness. His response, "You should consider writing up your experience in diabetes," planted the seed for this book. As the seed germinated, it evolved to focus on the patients' experiences rather than mine.

Several of our friends and family members reviewed all or part of the manuscript at various stages of its development and offered thoughtful critiques and suggestions. They include Frank Freemon, Steve Gabbe, Ginger Manley, Mayer Davidson, Rory and Rita Bourke, Susan Hales, Kim Emmons-Benjet, Ruthellen Sheldon, Edie Graber, Dean Graber, Lisa Graber Blain, and Susan Graber Schwabacher. Barbara Swift reviewed the manuscript word for word and offered extensive editing suggestions. To test the appropriateness of the book for a general audience, the members of Anne Brown's book club, the Fredericksburg Drive Readers, reviewed the manuscript as one of their monthly assignments, and many submitted written critiques.

The writers of several books influenced our efforts in using the narrative form to tell the stories of our patients. These include Studs Terkel, whose 1972 book, *Working*, portrayed the work of everyday Americans in their own words; Arthur Kleinman, author of *The Illness Narratives: Suffering, Healing, and the Human Condition* (1988); Anne Hunsaker Hawkins, author of *Reconstructing Illness: Studies in Pathography* (1999); Vivian Gornick, author of *The Situation and the Story: The Art of Personal Narratives* (2001); and Rita Charon, who published *Narrative Medicine: Honoring the Stories of Illness* (2006).

The little book *He Saw a Hummingbird,* by Norma Lee Browning and Russell Ogg, published in 1978, told us more about the development of blindness from diabetic retinopathy and the success in coping with this complication than any other written description of this disorder.

Fido's Coffee House, a few blocks from Vanderbilt Medical Center, served as our editorial office. In addition to serving superior coffee and breakfasts, the staff at Fido's, especially Khalil Davis and Jeff Gibbs, encouraged us like cheerleaders during the entire project.

Michael Ames, director of Vanderbilt University Press, encouraged us to pursue this book while it was still in its formative stage. His patience with rookie authors was extraordinary. His constant support and his repeated challenges to enhance the organization were the most significant forces in the book's development. In addition, he edited the entire manuscript and provided important suggestions for improvement.

Writing this book has reemphasized the importance of the support of our families. My wife, Edie, tolerated the sight of the back of my head in front of a computer screen for weeks at a time. Her critical reviews of several parts of the manuscript always stimulated and grounded my pondering. When I allowed myself to take too much poetic license in a few of the chapters, my son, Dean, a journalist, reminded me, "Dad, you're writing true accounts of patients' lives, not a novel." According to Anne and Kathleen, their patient and tolerant husbands, Larry Brown and Jim Price, respectively, did more than their share of household chores to enable them to work on this book. They also thank their parents and children, whose support and faith are unwavering.

Finally, we are grateful to the patients and their family members who shared their personal experiences for this book. In a larger sense, we are indebted to all the patients we have treated for all these years. They have entrusted us with the care of their health and with their lives, acts of trust that laid the foundation for this book. They have inspired us with their tenacity, with their courage, and with their resolute spirit in their struggles with diabetes. We respectfully dedicate this book to them.

ALG

Notes

PREFACE

1. M. Bliss, *The Discovery of Insulin* (Chicago: University of Chicago Press, 1982).
2. D. S. Ludwig, "Childhood obesity—the shape of things to come," *New England Journal of Medicine* 357 (2007): 2325–27.
3. S. H. Saydah, J. Fradkin, and C. C. Cowie, "Poor control of risk factors for vascular disease among adults with previously diagnosed diabetes," *Journal of the American Medical Association* 291 (2004): 335–42.
4. D. M. Nathan, J. Kuenen, R. Borg, H. Zheng, D. Schoenfeld, and J. J. Heine, for the A1c-derived average glucose (ADAG) study group, "Translating the A1c assay into estimated average glucose values," *Diabetes Care* 31 (2008): 1473–78.
5. American Diabetes Association, "Standards of Medical Care in Diabetes—2009," *Diabetes Care* 32, Supplement 1 (2009): S29.
6. Ibid., S30.

CHAPTER 5

1. H. A. Keenan, T. Costacou, J. K. Sun, et al., "Clinical factors associated with resistance to microvascular complications in diabetic patients of extreme disease duration: The 50-Year Medalist Study," *Diabetes Care* 30 (2007): 1995–97.
2. Department of Health and Human Services, "Autoimmune diseases and the promise of stem cell-based therapies," in *Regenerative Medicine*, August 2006, at *stemcells.nih.gov/info/2006report.htm*.

CHAPTER 7

1. American Diabetes Association, "Preconception care of women with diabetes," *Diabetes Care* 27 (2004), Supplement 1: S76–S78.

CHAPTER 8

1.   R. Charon, *Narrative Medicine: Honoring the Stories of Illness* (New York: Oxford University Press, 2006), 67.

CHAPTER 9

1.   "I asked for all things" comes from a text attributed to an unknown Confederate soldier.
2.   J. D. Piette and E. A. Kerr, "The impact of comorbid chronic conditions on diabetes care," *Diabetes Care* 29 (2006): 725–31.

PART II

1.   J. Solowiejczyk, "The family approach to diabetes management: Theory into practice toward the development of a new paradigm," *Diabetes Spectrum* 17 (2004): 31–36.

CHAPTER 11

1.   A. W. Frank, *The Wounded Storyteller* (Chicago: University of Chicago Press, 1995), 22.

CHAPTER 13

1.   H. P. Chase, "Nocturnal hypoglycemia—an unrelenting problem," *Journal of Clinical Endocrinology and Metabolism* 91 (2006): 2038–39.
2.   A. Kleinman, *The Illness Narratives: Suffering, Healing, and the Human Condition* (New York: Basic Books, 1988), 185.

CHAPTER 14

1.   Charon, *Narrative Medicine*, 75.

CHAPTER 16

1.   B. D. Metzger, T. A. Buchanan, D. R. Coustan, et al., "Summary and recommendations of the Fifth International Workshop-Conference on Gestational Diabetes Mellitus," *Diabetes Care* 30 (2007), Supplement 2: S251–S260.
2.   T. A. Buchanan, A. Xiang, S. L. Kjos, and R. Watanabe, "What is gestational diabetes?" *Diabetes Care* 30 (2007), Supplement 2: S105–S111.

CHAPTER 17

1. D. J. Cox, L. Gonder-Frederick, L. Ritterband, W. Clarke, and B. P. Kovatchev, "Prediction of severe hypoglycemia," *Diabetes Care* 30 (2007): 1370–73.
2. D. Deiss, J. Bolinder, J. Riveline, et al., "Improved glycemic control in poorly controlled patients with type 1 diabetes using real-time continuous glucose monitoring," *Diabetes Care* 29 (2006): 2730–32; T. S. Bailey, H. C. Zisser, and S. K. Garg, "Reduction in hemoglobin A1c with real-time continuous glucose monitoring: Results from a 12-week observational study," *Diabetes Technology and Therapeutics* 9 (2007): 203–10.

CHAPTER 18

1. K. Lim, A. Wilcox, M. Fisher, and C. I. Burns-Cox, "Type 1 diabetics and their pets," *Diabetic Medicine* 9 (1991): S3–S4; M. Chen, M. Daly, and G. Williams, "Non-invasive detection of hypoglycaemia using a novel, fully biocompatible, and patient friendly alarm system," *British Medical Journal* 321 (2000): 1655; D. L. Wells, S. W. Lawson, and A. N. Siriwardena, "Canine responses to hypoglycemia in patients with type 1 diabetes," *Journal of Alternative and Complementary Medicine* 14 (2008): 1177.
2. A. Spake, "Could a dog save your life?" *Diabetes Forecast*, March 2008.

CHAPTER 20

1. S. A. Morse, P. S. Ciechanowski, W. J. Katon, and I. B. Hirsch, "Isn't this just bedtime snacking? The potential adverse effects of night-eating symptoms on treatment adherence and outcomes in patients with diabetes," *Diabetes Care* 29 (2006): 1800–1804.
2. V. A. Fonseca, H. Smith, N. Kuhadiya, et al., "Impact of a Natural Disaster on Diabetes," *Diabetes Care* 32 (2009): 1632–38.

CHAPTER 21

1. ADA Statement: "Economic Costs of Diabetes in the U.S. in 2007," *Diabetes Care* 31 (2008): 596–615.

CHAPTER 23

1. M. Reiff, H. Zakut, and M. A. Weingarten, "Illness and treatment perceptions of Ethiopian immigrants and their doctors in Israel," *American Journal of Public Health* 89 (1999): 1814–18.
2. P. Hossain, B. Kawar, and M. El Nahas, "Obesity and diabetes in the developing world—a growing challenge," *New England Journal of Medicine* 356 (2007): 213–15.

CHAPTER 24

1. P. M. Just, F. T. deCharro, E. A. Tschosik, L. L. Noe, S. K. Bhattacharyya, and M. C. Riella, "Reimbursement and economic factors influencing dialysis modality choice around the world," *Nephrology Dialysis Transplantation* 23 (2008): 2365–73.

CHAPTER 26

1. Kleinman, *Illness Narratives*, 47.

PART IV

1. J. E. Aikens and J. D. Piette, "Diabetic patients' medication underuse, illness outcomes, and beliefs about antihyperglycemic and antihypertensive treatments," *Diabetes Care* 32 (2009): 19–24.
2. L. S. Phillips, W. T. Branch Jr., C. B. Cook, et al., "Clinical inertia," *Annals of Internal Medicine* 135 (2001): 825–34.
3. A. Larme and J. Pugh, "Attitudes of primary care providers toward diabetes: Barriers to guideline implementation," *Diabetes Care* 21 (1998): 1391–96.
4. T. B. Bodenheimer, "Primary care—will it survive?" *New England Journal of Medicine* 355 (2006): 861–64.
5. Charon, *Narrative Medicine*, 33.

CHAPTER 27

1. Diabetes Control and Complications Trial Research Group, "The effect of intensive treatment of diabetes on the development and progression of long term complications in insulin dependent diabetes mellitus," *New England Journal of Medicine* 329 (1993): 977–86.

CHAPTER 28

1. M. Heisler, S. Vijan, R. M. Anderson, P. A. Ubel, S. J. Benstein, and T. P. Hofer, "When do patients and their physicians agree on diabetes treatment goals and strategies, and what difference does it make?" *Journal of General Internal Medicine* 18 (2003): 893–902.

CHAPTER 29

1. D. J. Cox, L. A. Gonder-Frederick, B. P. Kovatchev, D. M. Julian, and W. L. Clarke, "Progressive hypoglycemia's impact on driving simulation performance: Occurrence, awareness, and correction," *Diabetes Care* 23 (2000): 163–70.

CHAPTER 30

1.   M. Peyrot, R. R. Rubin, T. Lauritzen, et al., on behalf of the international DAWN advisory panel, "Resistance to insulin therapy among patients and providers," *Diabetes Care* 28 (2005): 2673–79.
2.   M. C. Riddle, J. Rosenstock, and J. Gerich, on behalf of the Insulin Glargine 4002 Study Investigators, "The Treat-to-Target Trial: Randomized addition of glargine or human NPH insulin to oral therapy of type 2 diabetic patients," *Diabetes Care* 26 (2003): 3080–86.
3.   D. M. Nathan, J. B. Buse, M. B. Davidson, et al., "Management of hyperglycemia in type 2 diabetes: A consensus algorithm for the initiation and adjustment of therapy. A consensus statement from the American Diabetes Association and the European Association for the Study of Diabetes," *Diabetes Care* 29 (2006): 1963–72.
4.   S. Vijan, "The impact of diabetes on workforce participation: Results from a national household sample," *Health Services Research* 39 (2004): 1653–70.

CHAPTER 31

1.   American Diabetes Association, "Standards of Medical Care in Diabetes—2009," *Diabetes Care* 32 (2009), Supplement 1: S13–S61.

CHPTER 32

1.   A. Mohn, S. Di Michele, R. Di Luzio, S. Tumini, and F. Chiarelli, "The effect of subclinical hypothyroidism on metabolic control in children and adolescents with type 1 diabetes mellitus," *Diabetic Medicine* 19 (2002): 70–73.
2.   The Celiac Foundation, at *www.celiac.org*.

CHAPTER 33

1.   R. L. Rothman, R. Housam, H. Weiss, et al., "Patient understanding of food labels: The role of literacy and numeracy," *American Journal of Preventive Medicine* 20 (2006): 1–8; K. Cavanaugh, M. M. Huizenga, K. A. Wallston, et al., "Association of numeracy in diabetes control," *Annals of Internal Medicine* 148 (2006): 737–46; R. L. Rothman, V. M. Montori, A. Cherrington, and M. P. Pignone, "Perspective: The role of numeracy in health care," *Journal of Health Communication* 13 (2008): 583–95.

CHAPTER 34

1.   W. Katon, M. Von Korff, and P. Ciechanowski, "Behavioral and clinical factors associated with depression among individuals with diabetes," *Diabetes Care* 24 (2004): 1069–78.

2. W. J. Katon, G. Simon, and J. Russo, "Quality of depression care in a population-based sample of patients with diabetes and major depression," *Medical Care* 42 (2004): 1222–29.
3. R. B. Tattersall, "Psychiatric aspects of diabetes—a physician's view," *British Journal of Psychiatry* 139 (1981): 485–93.

CHAPTER 35

1. A. L. Graber, "Syndrome of lipodystrophy, hyperlipidemia, insulin resistance, and diabetes in treated patients with human immunodeficiency virus infection," *Endocrine Practice* 7 (2001): 430–37.

CONCLUSION

1. C. E. B. Couri, M. C. B. Oliveira, A. B. P. L. Stracieri, et al., "C-peptide levels and insulin independence following autologous nonmyeloablative hematopoietic stem cell transplantation in newly diagnosed type 1 diabetes mellitus," *Journal of the American Medical Association* 301 (2009): 1573–79.
2. S. Wild, G. Roglic, A. Green, R. Sicree, and H. King, "Global prevalence of diabetes: estimates for the year 2000 and projections for 2030," *Diabetes Care* 27 (2004): 1047–53.
3. W. C. Knowler, E. Barrett-Connor, S. E. Fowler, et al., "Reduction in the incidence of type 2 diabetes with lifestyle intervention or metformin," *New England Journal of Medicine* 346 (2002): 393–403.
4. X. R. Pan, G. W. Li, Y. H. Hu, et al., "Effects of diet and exercise in preventing NIDDM in people with impaired glucose tolerance: The Da Qing IGT and Diabetes Study," *Diabetes Care* 20 (1997): 537–44; J. Tuomilehto, J. Lindstrom, J. G. Eriksson, et al., "Prevention of type 2 diabetes mellitus by changes in lifestyle among subjects with impaired glucose tolerance," *New England Journal of Medicine* 344 (2001): 1343–50; A. Ramachandan, C. Snehalatha, S. May, B. Mukesh, A. D. Bhaskar, and V. Vijay, "The Indian Diabetes Prevention Programme shows that lifestyle modification and metformin prevent type 2 diabetes in Asian Indian subjects with impaired glucose tolerance (IDPP-1)," *Diabetologia* 49 (2006): 289–97.

Glossary

10 g filament. A small wire used to reproduce the amount of pressure that must be able to be felt to protect the foot from injury.

A1c. Average blood glucose. Normal individuals have A1c levels below 6 percent. A level above 6.5 percent is now considered diagnostic of diabetes. A1c is being increasingly reported as estimated average glucose (eAG): for example, an A1c of 5 percent is reported as 97 mg/dl, an A1c of 6 percent is reported as 126 mg/dl, and so on. For the prevention of microvascular disease (retinopathy, nephropathy, and neuropathy), the American Diabetes Association recommends an A1c goal for nonpregnant adults of below 7 percent. Less stringent goals may be appropriate for a patient with a history of severe hypoglycemia, limited life expectancy, advanced complications, or extensive comorbid conditions.

acute respiratory distress syndrome (ARDS). An illness which may last several weeks that affects the ability to get oxygen through lung tissue into the blood.

AIDS (acquired immunodeficiency syndrome). An illness caused by HIV in which the body's ability to fight infection is severely compromised.

albumin. A protein normally found in the blood but not normally found in the urine.

amputation. The surgical removal of a limb or part of a limb; for example, a toe or a leg.

angioplasty. The process of opening an artery by a "balloon" or a "coil" that is inserted by catheterization of the artery.

antihypertensive. A type of drug used to control high blood pressure.

ARDS. See **acute respiratory distress syndrome**.

arteriovenous shunt. A surgically created joining of an artery and a vein to provide easy access to the vascular system for hemodialysis.

autoimmune disorder. An illness caused by an attack of one's own immune cells on normal body tissues. In addition to type 1 diabetes, hypothyroidism, and celiac disease, other examples of autoimmune disease are Graves' disease (hyperthyroidism), rheumatoid arthritis, myasthenia gravis, lupus, and multiple sclerosis.

background retinopathy. See **diabetic eye disease**.

blood glucose. See **blood sugar**.

blood glucose monitoring. The process of checking blood sugar by a person at home, using a lancet to obtain a drop of blood and a small meter.

blood sugar. The level of glucose within the blood; normally less than 100 mg/dl before meals or 140 mg/dl two hours after meals in persons who do not have diabetes.

bolus. An extra dose of a drug; for example, an injection of insulin.

carbohydrate. A nutrient consisting of simple or complex sugars. Simple sugars, such as glucose or fructose, are found in sugar, honey, pancake syrup, fruit, fruit juice, soda drinks, and candy. Complex carbohydrates, sometimes called "starch," are present in foods such as bread, cereals, potatoes, pasta, and rice. Complex carbohydrates are digested to simple sugars in the bowel before absorption into the blood. The ingestion of carbohydrates results in transient elevation of blood sugar and prompts the secretion of insulin in individuals without diabetes. In persons with diabetes, the appropriate secretion of insulin is delayed and subnormal.

cardiovascular. Referring to the heart and the system of blood vessels throughout the body.

celiac disease. A condition in which the immune system responds abnormally to a protein called gluten, causing damage to the lining of the small intestine. Symptoms include diarrhea, malabsorption of many foods, and weight loss. Gluten is found in wheat, rye, barley, and many prepared foods.

certified diabetes educator (CDE). A registered nurse, dietitian, or other health professional who has specialized training in the care of people with diabetes, has a minimum of two years' experience caring for persons with diabetes, and has demonstrated evidence of their knowledge and expertise by passing a national certification exam.

closed loop. A type of insulin delivery system that would monitor blood glucose and respond by administering the correct amount of insulin from a pump or reservoir.

complication. An abnormality that develops in an organ of the body as the result of prolonged elevation of blood glucose, causing a loss of normal function.

compression stocking. Elastic stockings that provide pressure to the veins of the lower legs. Often used to prevent swelling, clots, or fall in blood pressure during standing.

congenital malformations (birth defects). Abnormalities present at birth. Many are minor, such as webbed toes, but serious ones could be fatal to the newborn, require surgical correction, or lead to marked physical or mental handicaps. In diabetes, these most commonly affect the cardiovascular system or the central nervous system.

congestive heart failure. A condition wherein the heart muscle is weakened, resulting in edema of the legs and congestion in the lungs.

control of blood sugar. Attempts to keep the blood glucose as close to the non-diabetes range as possible.

C-section or **cesarean section**. A surgical procedure to remove a baby from the uterus by making an incision through the abdomen and uterine wall.

diabetes. An ancient term referring to the process of water flowing through the body like a sieve. See also **diabetes mellitus** and **diabetes insipidus**.

diabetes insipidus. A much less frequent condition than diabetes mellitus, characterized by inability of the body to retain water, but with no abnormalities of blood glucose.

diabetes mellitus. A chronic disease characterized by elevated blood glucose levels. See also **type 1 diabetes**, **type 2 diabetes**, and **gestational diabetes**.

diabetes nurse educator. A registered nurse who has specialized knowledge and experience in the care and education of persons with diabetes; can be a certified diabetes educator if he or she passes an exam and meets other requirements.

diabetes nurse practitioner. A diabetes educator who also has a master's degree as a nurse practitioner. See also **nurse practitioner**.

diabetic. A person with diabetes mellitus.

diabetic eye disease (**retinopathy**). Changes in the small blood vessels of the retina, the light-sensitive rear lining of the eyeball. The first stage, called background retinopathy, consists of weakness and bulging of the retinal capillary walls. Background retinopathy, which causes no visual symptoms, can usually be detected by routine examination of the retina with an ophthalmoscope or by retinal photography. A more serious stage, called proliferative retinopathy, develops in a minority of those with background retinopathy. Fragile new blood vessels grow on the retinal surface and extend forward into the vitreous, potentially resulting in a vitreous hemorrhage.

diabetic ketoacidosis (**DKA**). An acute condition caused by a severe insulin deficiency, characterized by nausea, vomiting, dehydration, high blood sugar, presence of ketones in the blood and urine, and excess acid in the blood. If untreated, DKA can lead to coma and death.

diabetic kidney disease (**nephropathy**). A complication of diabetes caused by damage to the filtering system of the kidney. In its early stages, there is asymptomatic excretion of protein in the urine. If nephropathy is not treated successfully, it can result in kidney failure. Kidney failure is a fatal condition unless treated by dialysis or kidney transplant.

diabulimia. Purposely omitting insulin and using uncontrolled blood sugars to lose weight.

dialysis. A treatment used in kidney failure to replace the filtering process of the kidneys. See also **hemodialysis** and **peritoneal dialysis**.

dietitian. A health professional with specialized training in nutrition.

DKA. See **diabetic ketoacidosis**.

embryo. The early stages of the developing organism from the time of implantation in the womb through the eighth week after conception.

endocrinologist. A medical doctor who has completed an additional two to three years of training (after an internal medicine residency) in treating diseases of the endocrine glands, including diabetes.

endoscopy. An examination of the interior of a bodily canal or a hollow organ such as the colon, bladder, or stomach, using a slender, tubular optical instrument as a viewing system.

endothelium. The innermost lining of blood vessels. Abnormalities in the endothelium lead to narrowing and possibly occlusion of the blood vessels.

erectile dysfunction. Difficulty achieving or maintaining an erection suitable for coitus.

fasting blood sugar. The blood glucose level in the morning before breakfast, after no ingestion of food or beverages (except water) for eight to twelve hours.

fertilization. The union of a sperm and an egg.

fingerstick. Pricking of the fingertip with a sharp lancet to obtain a drop of blood for glucose measurement.

floaters. Abnormal specks in the field of vision of an eye. Most floaters are harmless and merely annoying, but in diabetes they may be an early indication of retinopathy.

footwear. See **therapeutic footwear**.

gestational diabetes (**GDM**). High blood sugar that first occurs during pregnancy.

glaucoma. Any of a group of eye diseases characterized by abnormally high intraocular fluid pressure. Glaucoma can lead to blindness. Glaucoma is more frequent in patients with diabetes.

glucagon. A hormone, normally produced by the alpha cells of the pancreas, which stimulates rapid glycogen breakdown to glucose in the liver and its release into the blood to increase blood glucose levels. It is available as an injection to treat severe hypoglycemia.

Glucophage. A pill used to treat type 2 diabetes. (The generic name is metformin.)

glucose. The sugar molecule normally found in the blood and body tissues. Glucose provides energy for body cells.

glucose monitor. A device about the size of a small cell phone used by persons to rapidly measure their blood glucose.

glucose tablets. Chewable tablets that provide four or five grams of glucose per tablet; used to treat low blood sugar.

glucose test strip. A chemically impregnated strip that measures blood sugar when a drop of blood is placed on it.

glucose tolerance test. A test used to diagnose diabetes or impaired glucose tolerance. After a fasting blood glucose specimen is obtained, the patient drinks 75 grams of a glucose-containing liquid. Subsequent blood glucose levels are measured at specific intervals for two hours.

glucosuria. The presence of glucose in the urine. Normally, no glucose is present in the urine.

Glucotrol. A pill that stimulates the secretion of insulin, used to treat type 2 diabetes. The generic name is glipizide.

gluten. A protein found in wheat, rye, and barley. Persons with celiac disease have an abnormal immune response to gluten.

glycosylated hemoglobin. The product of normal hemoglobin in the blood combining irreversibly with blood glucose. The level of glycosylated hemoglobin is proportional to the average blood glucose concentration over the preceding three or four months. See also **A1c**.

HDL. High-density lipoprotein, also known as "good" cholesterol.

hemodialysis (HD). A process of removing waste products from the blood by filtering it in a dialysis machine. The blood is derived from the arterial side of the circulation and returned to the venous side. The process takes about four hours, and in patients with chronic kidney failure is usually performed at a dialysis center three times a week.

hepatitis. Inflammation of the liver, caused by a virus or a toxin and characterized by jaundice, liver enlargement, and fever.

HIV (human immunodeficiency virus). The virus that causes AIDS.

home blood glucose monitoring. See **blood glucose monitoring**.

hypertension. High blood pressure. Although the diagnosis generally refers to a blood pressure greater than 140/90 in people without diabetes, the goal for treatment in patients with diabetes is less than 130/85.

hypoglycemia. Abnormally low blood glucose. When the blood sugar level is less than 70 mg/dl, symptoms such as nervousness, sweating, trembling, or rapid heart rate may occur. With lower levels, slowness in thinking, confusion, headache, and changes in vision may occur. At extremely low levels of blood glucose, confusion, stupor, loss of consciousness, or a seizure may occur.

hypoglycemic reaction. Presence of hypoglycemia; same as insulin reaction.

hypothyroidism. Deficient activity of the thyroid gland. At least 5 percent of patients with type 1 diabetes have hypothyroidism.

infusion set. The plastic tubing and small needle or plastic tube that connects the insulin reservoir of an insulin pump to the subcutaneous tissue (area under the skin) of the patient.

insulin. The hormone that allows glucose to enter body cells, normally secreted by the beta cells of the pancreatic islets. Its absence or deficiency causes diabetes.

insulin analogues. Synthetic types of insulin whose chemical structures have been altered slightly to change rate of absorption, onset of action, time of peak action, and duration of action.

insulin pen. A disposable or refillable penlike device that holds several doses of insulin.

insulin pump. A small, portable, battery-operated device usually worn on the belt. It contains a reservoir for a few days' supply of insulin and a tiny pump that propels the insulin outward at rates adjusted by the patient. The outlet of the insulin reservoir is connected to a fine plastic tube, the end of which is a tiny needle inserted under the skin (i.e., the infusion set). The insulin reservoir and the site of the needle insertion need to be changed every two or three days.

insulin reaction. The symptoms that occur as a result of an abnormally low blood sugar.

intensive insulin therapy. Taking multiple injections of insulin daily or using an insulin pump, along with frequent glucose monitoring, in an attempt to keep blood glucose close to normal levels.

interstitial fluid. The fluid between cells in the body tissues.

islet cells. The cells in the islets of Langerhans in the pancreas. The islet beta cells produce insulin.

islet cell transplant. An experimental procedure, currently available in only a few places. The pancreatic islets are extracted from the pancreas of someone who has just died. Then they are injected into the recipient, where they survive in the liver and secrete insulin.

IV glucose. Glucose administered through a vein (i.e., intravenously).

juvenile diabetes. A former term for type 1 diabetes. Though most cases of type 1 diabetes begin before age 20, type 1 diabetes can begin at any age.

LADA (latent autoimmune diabetes of adults). A term used to describe atypical cases of type 1 diabetes that develop in adulthood. The clinical appearance is usually more typical of type 2 diabetes, because it develops gradually and insidiously, often without symptoms, and therefore is usually initially diagnosed as type 2 diabetes. Insulin treatment is often not necessary, at least at the onset. However, low levels of antibodies directed at the islet cells of the pancreas are present, indicating an autoimmune cause rather than one related to obesity, insulin resistance, or lifestyle.

lancet. A small blade used for making a puncture in a fingertip to obtain a drop of blood.

Lantus. An insulin analogue that provides a steady level of insulin in the body for about twenty-four hours.

laparoscopic. Referring to a procedure using a laparoscope, a slender, flexible fiber-optic instrument used to examine the abdominal or pelvic cavity. Inserted through a small incision in the abdominal wall, a laparoscope can be used to perform a biopsy or surgery. Laparoscopic surgery is often referred to as "Band-Aid" surgery because it requires only small incisions.

laser therapy. A laser is a device that generates a concentrated beam of light. The heat from this light is used to treat diabetic retinopathy. See also **panretinal photocoagulation** and **macular edema**.

latent autoimmune diabetes of adults. See **LADA**.

LDL. Low-density lipoprotein, also known as "bad" cholesterol.

lipid-lowering drugs. The category of drugs that decrease cholesterol or triglyceride levels.

lipid profile. A blood test that measures total cholesterol, the LDL and HDL cholesterol fractions, and triglycerides. The blood sample must be obtained in the fasting state before breakfast.

low blood sugar. Hypoglycemia, or blood sugar level below 70 mg/dl.

macrosomia. An abnormally large infant, usually referring to a newborn weighing ten pounds or more. Macrosomia can be a complication of both gestational diabetes and pregnancy in a woman with preexisting diabetes.

macular edema. A condition of blurred vision caused by leakage of fluid from the small blood vessels around the macula, the area of sharpest vision in the retina. This condition is sometimes treated by focal laser photocoagulation.

malabsorption. A decrease of absorption of nutrients and vitamins from the intestine.

metabolic syndrome. A cluster of common abnormalities characterized by increased waist circumference, elevated triglycerides, low HDL, high blood pressure, and sometimes by borderline or elevated blood sugar. It carries an increased risk of diabetes and of cardiovascular disease.

metformin. A drug commonly used to treat type 2 diabetes. Metformin acts by decreasing production of glucose by the liver, not by increasing insulin secretion.

mg/dl. Milligrams per deciliter; the unit of measurement used to quantify the concentration of glucose or other chemicals in the blood.

microalbuminuria. Very small amounts of protein in the urine that indicate early kidney damage from high blood sugar. The low concentration of albumin is not found in a routine urinalysis but requires a special test for its detection. It is commonly reported as the microalbumin/creatinine ratio.

neuropathy. Diabetes complication that occurs when nerves are damaged by high blood sugar.

nocturnal hypoglycemia. Subnormal blood glucose levels occurring at night, often unrecognized.

nurse practitioner. A registered nurse who has obtained a master's degree in nursing, has received advanced training in the diagnosis and treatment of human illness, and has the authority to prescribe medication. Nurse practitioners may also hold certification in advanced diabetes management, which requires additional experience and training. See also **diabetes nurse practitioner**.

orthostatic hypotension. A condition in which the blood pressure falls when the person stands. Sometimes the fall in blood pressure causes lightheadedness or fainting.

panretinal photocoagulation. A procedure in which a high-energy source of light produces a small burn of the retina. When proliferative retinopathy is present, thousands of small burns are placed around the periphery of the retina, reducing the proliferation of abnormal blood vessels. This procedure reduces the risk of sight-threatening vitreous hemorrhage and blindness. See also **diabetic eye disease**.

pathologist. A medical specialist who examines samples of body tissues for diagnostic purposes.

perimenopausal. The years during which the transition into menopause is occurring but menstrual cycles may not have ceased.

peritoneal dialysis (PD). A treatment for kidney failure. The process uses the surface of the abdominal cavity (the peritoneum) as a membrane through which fluid and molecules are exchanged with the blood. Fluid is introduced into the abdomen through a tube. During the time the fluid dwells in the abdomen, it accumulates waste products that ordinarily would be excreted by the kidneys. Then the fluid is removed via the tube, and the process is repeated. Usually this procedure is performed at night while the patient sleeps.

phantom pain. The sensation of pain perceived to exist in a limb that has been amputated.

post-prandial blood glucose. The blood glucose level after a meal.

pre-diabetes. A condition with blood glucose levels higher than normal but not high enough to meet diagnostic criteria for diabetes. Normal fasting plasma glucose level is less than 100 mg/dl. A fasting plasma glucose level above 125 mg/dl indicates the presence of diabetes. Impaired fasting glucose is therefore defined as fasting plasma glucose level between 100 and 125 mg/dl. Likewise, two hours after an individual drinks 75 grams of glucose during a glucose tolerance test, normal plasma glucose concentration is less than 140 mg/dl, and diabetes is present if the two-hour plasma glucose concentration is 200 mg/dl or greater. Impaired glucose tolerance is thus defined as a two-hour plasma glucose concentration between 140 and 200 mg/dl. Some individuals with pre-diabetes have isolated impaired fasting glucose; others have isolated impaired glucose tolerance, and many have a combination of the two abnormalities.

pre-eclampsia. See **toxemia**.

proliferative diabetic retinopathy. See **diabetic eye disease**.

prosthesis. An artificial device replacing a missing part of the body.

protease inhibitors. A group of drugs used to inhibit the growth of certain viruses. Commonly used to treat HIV and AIDS.

retina. The light-sensitive inner lining of the rear of the rear of the eyeball where images from the lens are projected. The retina is connected by the optic nerve to the brain.

retinopathy. See **diabetic eye disease**.

sleep apnea. A common disorder, especially in obese persons, characterized by episodes of interrupted breathing during sleep, not remembered by the patient. Those suffering from severe sleep apnea typically complain of sleepiness, irritability, forgetfulness, and difficulty in concentrating.

Splenda. Brand name for an artificial sweetener containing sucralose. Sucralose is sweeter than sucrose (table sugar), saccharin, and aspartame.

staph infection. An infection caused by the staphylococcus bacteria.

statin. A class of medication used to decrease cholesterol levels.

syringe. A device used to inject medication with a needle.

therapeutic footwear. Footwear designed to protect the foot from injury or to accommodate deformities in the foot.

toxemia. An abnormal condition of pregnancy characterized by hypertension, fluid retention, edema, and the presence of protein in the urine. The modern term is pre-eclampsia. Severe cases with coma or convulsions are called eclampsia.

TrialNet. An international network of clinical centers that provide screening for family members of patients with type 1 diabetes, in order to identify persons at risk for development of type 1 diabetes. TrialNet offers studies to prevent type 1 diabetes in persons at risk and studies to slow its progression in patients recently diagnosed with type 1 diabetes. More information is available at *www.diabetestrialnet.org*.

triglyceride. One of the fats normally circulating in the blood, containing three fatty acids linked to glycerol. Triglycerides are also the main component of adipose tissue.

trimester. Any of three periods of approximately three months each into which a human pregnancy is divided.

type 1 diabetes. See the Preface.

type 2 diabetes. See the Preface.

ulcer. An open sore or break in the skin. In the foot of a person with diabetes, an ulcer is usually caused by unrecognized pressure from a shoe.

unit. The measurement used for insulin doses. Units are used because insulin is used in such small amounts that it cannot be safely measured in the more standard milliliters. Most commonly, one hundred units equal one milliliter. More concentrated forms of insulin containing five hundred units per milliliter are also available for patients requiring large insulin doses.

vascular. Relating to blood vessels.

villi. Small fingerlike structures normally lining the small intestine that absorb nutrients. The villi become flattened in people with celiac disease. Once gluten is removed from the diet, the villi resume a normal pattern.

vitrectomy. Surgical removal of the vitreous in an attempt to restore vision after a vitreous hemorrhage has occurred.

vitreous. The jellylike center of the eyeball.

vitreous hemorrhage. The rupture of an abnormal retinal blood vessel into the eyeball. The hemorrhage blocks light rays from reaching the retina. When light does not reach the retina, no visual image is formed, and loss of vision results.

Internet Resources for Patients with Diabetes

The American Association of Diabetes Educators (AADE) is an organization of health care professionals that aims to "promote healthy living through self-management of diabetes." The Web site has links to local diabetes educators, resources for patients, and a blog authored by diabetes educators who are members of AADE. The blog allows visitors to engage in conversations about their experiences.
www.DiabetesEducator.org

The American Diabetes Association (ADA) has a mission "to prevent and cure diabetes and to improve the lives of all people affected by diabetes." The ADA fights "against the deadly consequences of diabetes and fights for those affected by diabetes." The Web site has links to resources for living with diabetes and monitored chat rooms. In addition, one can obtain information in Spanish.
www.Diabetes.org

The Behavioral Diabetes Institute is a nonprofit organization "dedicated to tackling the unmet psychological needs of people with diabetes."
www.BehavioralDiabetesInstitute.org

The Centers for Disease Control and Prevention (CDC) works "to eliminate the preventable burden of diabetes through leadership, research, programs, and policies." CDC's Division of Diabetes Translation "translates diabetes research into daily practice to understand the impact of the disease, influence health outcomes, and improve access to quality health care." The Web site provides information about diabetes, including research, statistics, and educational publications.
www.CDC.gov/diabetes

Diabetes Forecast, the consumer magazine published by the ADA, publishes an annual Consumer Guide, which evaluates diabetes products such as blood glucose meters, continuous glucose monitors, insulin pumps and infusion sets,

insulin pens, and other products, including products not yet introduced on the market. It also offers news on diabetes research and treatment and provides information, inspiration, and support to people with diabetes.
www.Forecast.Diabetes.org

DiabetesHealth is an electronic newsletter with links to numerous diabetes product reference guides.
www.DiabetesHealth.com/charts

Diabetes Self-Management publishes a bimonthly magazine, a weekly e-mail newsletter, a number of books, and a blog. The magazine offers information on nutrition, exercise, new drugs, medical advances, and self-help.
www.DiabetesSelfManagement.com

The Juvenile Diabetes Research Foundation (JDRF) seeks "a cure for diabetes and its complications through the support of research. . . . Since its founding in 1970 by parents of children with type 1 diabetes, JDRF has awarded more than $1 billion to diabetes research, including more than $1 million in FY2009." The Web site offers support, research, advocacy, and other resources.
www.jdrf.org

Mendosa.com, a Web site that catalogs 250 online resources for diabetes, is maintained by a freelance medical writer.
www.Mendosa.com

The National Diabetes Information Clearinghouse (NDIC) is an information dissemination service of the National Institute of Diabetes and Digestive and Kidney Diseases (NIDDK).
diabetes.niddk.nih.gov

Taking Control of Your Diabetes (TCOYD) conferences and health fairs around the nation provide information on clinical research, the emergence of new equipment and medications, proper diet and exercise, and legal and insurance issues, as well as offering other resources.
Tcoyd.org

TrialNet is "an international network of researchers who are exploring ways to prevent, delay and reverse the progression of type 1 diabetes." The Web site provides links to regional clinical centers so that individuals can find the nearest of the two hundred locations that participate in screening and clinical studies. Studies are also available for family members of persons with type 1 diabetes.
www.DiabetesTrialNet.org

Reader's Guide to Topics

Work issues

Visual impairment

Index

Page numbers in bold refer to photos.